ENDOLEAKS

&

ENDOTENSION

ENDOLEAKS & ENDOTENSION

Current Consensus on Their Nature and Significance

edited by

Frank J. Veith

Montefiore Medical Center–
Albert Einstein College of Medicine
New York, New York, U.S.A.

Richard A. Baum

Brigham & Women's Hospital
and *Harvard Medical School*
Boston, Massachusetts, U.S.A.

informa

healthcare

New York London

First published in 2003 by Marcel Dekker, Inc.

This edition published in 2010 by Informa Healthcare, Telephone House, 69-77 Paul Street, London EC2A 4LQ, UK.

Simultaneously published in the USA by Informa Healthcare, 52 Vanderbilt Avenue, 7th Floor, New York, NY 10017, USA.

Informa Healthcare is a trading division of Informa UK Ltd. Registered Office: 37–41 Mortimer Street, London W1T 3JH, UK. Registered in England and Wales number 1072954.

A CIP record for this book is available from the British Library.

Library of Congress Cataloging-in-Publication Data available on application

ISBN-13: 9780824709549

Orders may be sent to: Informa Healthcare, Sheepen Place, Colchester, Essex CO3 3LP, UK
Telephone: +44 (0)20 7017 5540
Email: CSDhealthcarebooks@informa.com
Website: http://informahealthcarebooks.com/

For corporate sales please contact: CorporateBooksIHC@informa.com
For foreign rights please contact: RightsIHC@informa.com
For reprint permissions please contact: PermissionsIHC@informa.com

Preface

Like other new endoluminal treatments, endovascular aortic aneurysm repair (EVAR) has generated a great deal of interest—and, along with it, considerable controversy. Some of this controversy surrounds the complications of EVAR and what to do about them. Resolving these contentious issues is becoming more important because as the endografts remain in place for longer periods of time, the incidence of problems is increasing.

Clearly, the most common problems developing after EVAR are the occurrence of endoleaks (blood flow outside the graft) and endotension (increased pressure within the aneurysm sac). Although all will agree that these entities have a complex etiology, there is much disagreement about how best to diagnose and manage them when they occur.

We conceived of the William J. von Liebig Consensus Conferences in 1999 as a way to clear confusion, resolve disagreement, and/or provide an overview of the state of knowledge and opinion regarding an unclear or controversial topic in an emerging endovascular treatment modality. Certainly the nature and significance of endoleaks and endotension are ideal topics to address through such a consensus process. These problems, and what to do for the patients who have them, present an increasing challenge to those involved in EVAR. Moreover, we need to do a better job of preventing them.

In late 2000, 27 experienced experts with a profound interest in endoleaks and endotension came together to focus on these topics. This book represents a distillate of their consensus process and its conclusions. It also includes chapters by these experts. Each chapter presents relevant data and individual perspectives and opinions.

Although answers to all questions regarding endoleaks and endotension may not be known, this volume summarizes the current state of knowledge and opinion regarding these problems. It will serve as a guide to management and a starting point for those interested in advancing knowledge about endoleaks and endotension and what to do to prevent and treat them more effectively.

Frank J. Veith
Richard A. Baum

Contents

Contents

Contributors

Mohan Adiseshiah, F.R.C.P., F.R.C.S. Consultant, Vascular/Endovascular Surgery, Vascular Unit, University College London Hospital, London, England

John L. Anderson, F.A.C.S., F.R.A.C.S. Ashford Hospital, Adelaide, South Australia, Australia

Richard A. Baum, M.D. Herbert L. Abrams Director of Angiography and Interventional Radiology, Department of Radiology, Brigham & Women's Hospital, and Harvard Medical School, Boston, Massachusetts, U.S.A.

Jan D. Blankensteijn, M.D. Associate Professor, Department of Vascular Surgery, University Medical Center Utrecht, Utrecht, The Netherlands

Jacob Buth, M.D. Consulting Vascular Surgeon, Department of Surgery, Catharina Hospital, Eindhoven, The Netherlands

Timothy A. M. Chuter, D.M. Associate Professor in Residence, Department of Surgery, and Director, Endovascular Surgery Program, University of California at San Francisco, San Francisco, California, U.S.A.

Miguel A. Cuesta, M.D.   Chief, Division of Minimally Invasive Surgery, and Professor, Department of Surgery, Vrije University, and Vrije University Medical Center, Amsterdam, The Netherlands

Carlos Donayre, M.D.   Division of Vascular Surgery, Department of Surgery, Harbor-UCLA Medical Center, Torrance, California, U.S.A.

Ronald M. Fairman, M.D.   Associate Professor, Departments of Surgery and Radiology, and Chief, Division of Vascular Surgery, Department of Surgery, University of Pennsylvania School of Medicine, and University of Pennsylvania Medical Center, Philadelphia, Pennsylvania, U.S.A.

Luis Mariano Ferreira, M.D.   Department of Vascular Surgery, Cardiovascular Institute of Buenos Aires, Buenos Aires, Argentina

Geoffrey L. Gilling-Smith, M.S., F.R.C.S.   Senior Lecturer in Surgery, University of Liverpool, and Consultant Vascular Surgeon, Regional Vascular Unit, Royal Liverpool University Hospital, Liverpool, England

NavYash Gupta, M.D.   Assistant Professor, Division of Vascular Surgery, Department of Surgery, University of Pittsburgh Medical Center, and Presbyterian University Hospital, Pittsburgh, Pennsylvania, U.S.A.

Peter Lyon Harris, M.D., F.R.C.S.   Department of Surgery, University of Liverpool, and Clinical Director, Vascular Surgical Services, Department of Surgery, Royal Liverpool University Hospital, Liverpool, England

Robert J. Hinchliffe, M.R.C.S.   Research Fellow, Departments of Vascular and Endovascular Surgery, University Hospital, Nottingham, England

Kim J. Hodgson, M.D.   Professor and Chairman, Division of Vascular Surgery, Department of Surgery, Southern Illinois University School of Medicine, Springfield, Illinois, U.S.A.

Brian R. Hopkinson, M.B., Ch.M., F.R.C.S.   Professor, Department of Vascular Surgery, University of Nottingham, and University Hospital, Nottingham, England

Krassi Ivancev, M.D. Associate Professor, Department of Diagnostic Radiology, Lund University, and Chief, Endovascular Center, Department of Diagnostic Radiology, Malmö University Hospital, Malmö, Sweden

Michael M. D. Lawrence-Brown, F.R.A.C.S. Emeritus Consultant, Department of Vascular Surgery, Royal Perth Hospital, Perth, Western Australia, Australia

Christopher J. LeSar, M.D. Clinical Vascular Fellow, Division of Vascular Surgery, Department of Surgery, Eastern Virginia Medical School, Norfolk, Virginia, U.S.A.

Michel S. Makaroun, M.D. Professor, Division of Vascular Surgery, Department of Surgery, University of Pittsburgh Medical Center, and Presbyterian University Hospital, Pittsburgh, Pennsylvania, U.S.A.

Martin Malina, M.D., Ph.D. Associate Professor, Department of Vascular Surgery, Lund University, and Department of Vascular Diseases and Endovascular Center, Malmö University Hospital, Malmö, Sweden

James May, M.D., F.R.A.C.S., F.A.C.S. Bosch Professor, Department of Surgery, University of Sydney, and Royal Prince Alfred Hospital, Sydney, New South Wales, Australia

George H. Meier, M.D., F.A.C.S. Chief, Division of Vascular Surgery, Department of Surgery, Eastern Virginia Medical School, and Norfolk Surgical Group Ltd., Norfolk, Virginia, U.S.A.

Takao Ohki, M.D. Chief, Division of Vascular Surgery, Department of Surgery, Montefiore Medical Center–Albert Einstein College of Medicine, New York, New York, U.S.A.

Juan Carlos Parodi, M.D. Vice Director, Post-Graduate Training Program in Cardiovascular Surgery, University of Buenos Aires, and Chief, Department of Cardiovascular Surgery, Cardiovascular Institute of Buenos Aires, Buenos Aires, Argentina

Jan A. Rauwerda, M.D., Ph.D. Professor and Chief, Department of Surgery, Vrije University, and Vrije University Medical Center, Amsterdam, The Netherlands

Timothy Resch, M.D.   Fellow, Department of Surgery, Malmö University Hospital, Malmö, Sweden

Abraham Rijbroek, M.D.   Department of Surgery, Vrije University, and Vrije University Medical Center, Amsterdam, The Netherlands

James B. Semmens, Ph.D.   Director, Centre for Health Services Research, School of Population Health, University of Western Australia, Nedlands, Western Australia, Australia

Maurice M. Solis, M.D., F.A.C.S.   Chief, Division of Vascular and Endovascular Surgery, Department of Surgery, Macon Cardio-Vascular Institute, Macon, Georgia, U.S.A.

Björn Sonesson, M.D.   Associate Professor, Department of Surgery, Lund University, and Department of Vascular Diseases and Endovascular Center, Malmö University Hospital, Malmö, Sweden

S. William Stavropoulos, M.D.   Assistant Professor, Departments of Radiology and Surgery, University of Pennsylvania School of Medicine, and University of Pennsylvania Medical Center, Philadelphia, Pennsylvania, U.S.A.

Frank J. Veith, M.D.   Professor and Vice Chairman, Department of Surgery, and William J. von Liebig Chair in Vascular Surgery, Montefiore Medical Center–Albert Einstein College of Medicine, New York, New York, U.S.A.

Omaida C. Velazquez, M.D.   Assistant Professor, Division of Vascular Surgery, John Rhea Barton Department of Surgery, University of Pennsylvania School of Medicine, and University of Pennsylvania Medical Center, Philadelphia, Pennsylvania, U.S.A.

Irwin Walot, M.D.   Division of Vascular Surgery, Department of Surgery, Harbor-UCLA Medical Center, Torrance, California, U.S.A.

Geoffrey H. White, M.D.   Associate Professor, Endovascular Research Unit, Department of Surgery, University of Sydney, and Royal Prince Alfred Hospital, Sydney, New South Wales, Australia

Rodney A. White, M.D. Chief, Division of Vascular Surgery, Department of Surgery, Harbor-UCLA Medical Center, Torrance, California, U.S.A.

Willem Wisselink, M.D., PhD. Associate Professor, Department of Surgery, Vrije University, and Vrije University Medical Center, Amsterdam, The Netherlands

Christopher K. Zarins, M.D. Chidester Professor, Division of Vascular Surgery, Department of Surgery, Stanford University, Stanford, California, U.S.A.

1

Introduction and Methods

Frank J. Veith
Montefiore Medical Center–Albert Einstein College of Medicine, New York, New York, U.S.A.

Richard A. Baum
Brigham & Women's Hospital and Harvard Medical School, Boston, Massachusetts, U.S.A.

Endovascular abdominal aortic aneurysm repair (EVAR) has been performed since 1990 (1). A variety of endograft devices have been used at centers around the world (2–6). Although many dramatically successful early results have been achieved and many advantages are claimed, the mid- and long-term durability of these grafts and their effectiveness in preventing rupture remain questionable (7–10). One of the principal reasons for failure after the first year is the occurrence of *endoleaks*, defined as persistent blood flow outside the graft and within the aneurysm sac (11). Another reason is the presence of *endotension*, defined as a state of elevated pressure within the aneurysm sac (12).

It is generally agreed that endoleaks and endotension are critically important complications of many EVARs. However, many aspects of the nature, incidence, and significance of these problems are highly controversial. Some believe that most endoleaks do not influence the outcome of EVARs (13), whereas others consider most of them to be serious and regard them as the Achilles heel of the procedure (10,11). In addition, wide differences of opinion exist regarding how best to treat endoleaks and endotension. Even the classification systems for these problems and the relationship between them remain subjects of controversy (14,15).

1

Table 1.   Consensus Participants

Vascular surgeons	Interventional radiologists	Interventional cardiologists
Adiseshiah, Mohan	Baum, Richard A.	Amor, Max
Blankensteijn, Jan D.	Ivancev, Krassi	
Buth, Jacob	Katzen, Barry T.	
Chuter, Timothy A. M.	Richter, Götz M.	
Fairman, Ronald M.	Rubin, Geoffrey D.[a]	
Gilling-Smith, Geoffrey L.		
Harris, Peter Lyon		
Hodgson, Kim J.		
Hopkinson, Brian R.		
Lawrence-Brown, Michael M. D.		
Makaroun, Michel S.		
Malina, Martin		
Meier, George H.		
Ohki, Takao		
Parodi, Juan Carlos		
Stelter, Wolf J.		
Veith, Frank J.		
White, Geoffrey H.		
White, Rodney A.		
Wisselink, Willem		
Zarins, Christopher K.		

[a] An expert in vascular imaging.

To resolve some of these controversies and the conflicting recommendations for management related to endoleaks and endotension, it was decided to hold a conference of world opinion leaders on these topics. The main purpose of this consensus conference, which included experts from several disciplines interested in EVAR, was to reach agreement or consensus on as many key issues related to endoleaks and endotension as possible. A second purpose was to define areas of uncertainty or unanswered questions regarding these two entities. The present book summarizes the results of this consensus-seeking process and provides an overview of the current state of knowledge concerning endoleaks and endotension. This information should be helpful in guiding patient-management decisions. It may also prove useful in evaluating the overall effectiveness of EVAR and in guiding future investigations relating to these two important complications.

I. METHODS

To provide the most informed yet balanced overview of the endoleak/endo-tension field, the consensus conference organizers (FJV, RAB) selected as participants individuals who were generally acknowledged as leaders in the field, i.e., those physicians who, irrespective of the specialty they represented, had the widest experience and greatest interest in endoleaks and endotension and who had studied these processes and published most extensively on them. Twenty-seven participants were chosen from three different specialties (vascular surgery, interventional radiology, and interventional cardiology) and nine different countries (United States, United Kingdom, France, Germany, Denmark, Sweden, Australia, Argentina, and the Netherlands). As shown in Table 1, 21 of these participants were vascular surgeons, 4 were interventional radiologists, 1 was an expert in vascular imaging techniques, and 1 was an interventional, cardiologist. All 27 of the participants had extensive experience in performing EVAR and/or evaluating EVAR patients before and/or after their procedures. All had lectured and written widely about the diagnoses and/or management of endoleaks and endotension. All the selected participants agreed to take part in the consensus process and its subsequent documentation.

II. BEFORE THE ORAL CONSENSUS CONFERENCE

All participants were sent a questionnaire requesting their responses to 40 key questions relating to endoleaks and endotension. These questions related to the timing, incidence, nature of endoleaks and endotension, how they should be classified, how they should be diagnosed and managed, and how they are related to each other and to the outcomes of EVAR. These questions were designed to evaluate current points of agreement or disagreement about various critical issues regarding these complications. The answers to these questions plus discussion of both the questions and answers at the oral session would serve as the major basis for the written documentation that would be the product of the consensus process. The questionnaire had room for comments in addition to the "agree," "disagree," or "uncertain" answers or percentage answers that were possible for most of the questions. Twenty-six of the participants returned their completed questionnaire in time for the answers to be collated and analyzed before the oral session. Thus, answers and questions could be discussed effectively at the oral session.

III. ORAL CONSENSUS CONFERENCE

This conference was held in New York City on November 20, 2000. Five of the 27 participants were unable to attend because of prior commitments or urgent conflicts. The views of 2 of these 5 were represented by colleagues who did attend (Peter Harris for Geoffrey Gilling-Smith and Christopher Zarins for Geoffrey Rubin). An audience of approximately 100 interested physicians also attended the conference and participated in the discussion.

The oral session consisted of a short introductory statement outlining the purpose and structure of the session and the documentation that would result. A summary and analysis of the participants' answers to each of the 40 original questions was then presented. Discussion of each question and its answers followed. Two questions were modified slightly to permit answers to which most participants could agree. In other instances participants' answers were changed as the question was clarified by the discussion. An effort was made by all to reach consensus or near-consensus on as many of the answers as possible within the limits of participants' experience and opinions. Free discussion of each question of and issue was encouraged, and then a summary statement was made regarding each. All discussion was recorded for subsequent review by the conference organizers so that important facts and opinions could be included in the conference documentation. A major goal of all present was to resolve areas of disagreement, if possible, and if not, to clarify the areas of residual disagreement.

IV. WRITTEN DOCUMENTATION OF THE CONSENSUS PROCESS

This volume serves as the primary documentation of the consensus process. The next chapter summarizes the participants' answers to the 40 questions originally posed as well as the 2 modified questions arrived at during the oral conference discussion. Based on the these answers and the accompanying comments and discussion, the next two chapters will also provide a broad consensus and prevailing opinion overview summarizing current thinking regarding endoleaks and endotension. It will also highlight areas of uncertainty and directions for future investigation.

In addition to these first three chapters, other chapters from most of the consensus participants are included, all of whom have been asked to detail their views, experience, and predictions regarding endoleaks and endotension.

REFERENCES

1. Parodi JC, Palmaz JC, Barone HD. Transfemoral intraluminal graft implantation for abdominal aortic aneurysms. Ann Vasc Surg 1991; 5:491–499.
2. Moore WS. The EVT tube and bifurcated graft systems: technical considerations and clinical summary. J Endovasc Surg 1997; 4:182–194.
3. Marin ML, Veith FJ, Cynamon J, Sanchez LA, et al. Initial experience with transluminally placed endovascular grafts for the treatment of complex vascular lesions. Ann Surg 1995; 222:449–469.
4. Blum U, Voshage G, Lammer J, et al. Endoluminal stent-grafts for infrarenal abdominal aortic aneurysms. N Engl J Med 1997; 336:13–20.
5. Zarins CK, White RA, Schwarten D, et al. AneuRx stent graft versus open surgical repair of abdominal aortic aneurysms: multicenter prospective clinical trial. J Vasc Surg 1999; 29(2):292–308.
6. Criado FJ, Wilson EP, Fairman RM, Abul-Khoudoud O, Wellons E. Update on the Talent aortic stent-graft: a preliminary report from United States phase I and II trials. J Vasc Surg 2001; 33(2 suppl):S146–149.
7. Zarins CK, White RA, Fogarty TJ. Aneurysm rupture after endovascular repair using the AneuRx stent graft. J Vasc Surg 2000; 31(5):960–970.
8. Holzbein TJ, Kretschmer G, Thurnher S, et al. Midterm durability of abdominal aortic aneurysm endograft repair: a word of caution. J Vasc Surg 2001; 33(2 Pt 2):46–54.
9. Harris PL, Vallabhaneni SR, Desgranges P, et al. Incidence and risk factors of late rupture, conversion, and death after endovascular repair of infrarenal aortic aneurysms: the EUROSTAR experience. European collaborators on stent/graft techniques for aortic aneurysm repair. J Vasc Surg 2000; 32(4):739–749.
10. Ohki T, Veith FJ, Shaw P, et al. Increasing incidence of mid and long-term complications after endovascular graft repair of AAAs: a note of caution based on a 9-year experience. Ann Surg 2001; 234:323–335.
11. White GH, Yu W, May J, et al. Endoleaks as a complication of endoluminal grafting of abdominal aortic aneurysms: classification, incidence, diagnosis, and management. J Endovasc Surg 1997; 4:152–168.
12. Gilling-Smith GL, Brennan J, Harris P, et al. Endotension after endovascular aneurysm repair: definition, classification, and strategies for surveillance and intervention. J Endovasc Surg 1999; 6:305–307.
13. Zarins CK, White RA, Hodgson KJ, et al. Endoleak as a predictor of outcome after endovascular aneurysm repair: AneuRx multicenter clinical trial. J Vasc Surg 2000; 32:90–107.
14. Gilling-Smith GL, Harris PL, McWilliams RG. How should endotension be defined? J Endovasc Ther 2000; 7:439–440.
15. White GH, May J. How should endotension be defined? History of a concept and evolution of a new term. J Endovasc Ther 2000; 7:435–438.

2

Results of Consensus Questionnaire and Conference Process

Frank J. Veith
Montefiore Medical Center–Albert Einstein College of Medicine, New York, New York, U.S.A.

Richard A. Baum
Brigham & Women's Hospital and Harvard Medical School, Boston, Massachusetts, U.S.A.

I. DEFINITIONS

Answers to all 42 questions were analyzed and interpreted according to the definitions shown in Table 1. If 18 or more of the 26 responding participants agreed on a response to a question, that answer was considered to represent consensus or general agreement. If 14–17 of the 26 respondents agreed, that response was considered to represent near-consensus or prevailing opinion. If fewer than 14 of the 26 participants agreed on a response to a question, that response was considered an area of divided opinion, disagreement, or uncertainty.

II. RESULTS OF CONSENSUS QUESTIONNAIRE AND CONFERENCE

A. Overall Results

Of the 40 questions originally posed to the conference participants, consensus or agreement with regard to the answer was attained on 22 and near-consensus

Table 1.   Interpretation of Answers by 26 Participating Experts

Consistent answers	Interpretation/definition
≥ 18/26	Consensus (agreement)
14–17/26	Prevailing opinion (near-consensus)
< 14/26	Divided opinion/disagreement (uncertainty)

or prevailing opinion on an additional 14. The answers to the 4 remaining original questions reflected divided opinion or wide ranges of opinion, based on conflicting views, uncertainty, or actual disagreement. In addition, at the oral conference two derivative or altered questions were posed. With these modified questions, the answers were converted from prevailing opinion to consensus. Thus, consensus was reached on 24 of 42 or 57% of the answers to key questions posed, and near-consensus was reached on 14 of 42 or 33% of the answers. Only with the answers to 4 of the 42 or 10% of the questions was there a wide range of divergent opinions. These overall results reflect a remarkable degree of agreement among the experts on these controversial and perplexing topics.

B. Consensus or General Agreement Results

Consensus Relating to Nature or Behavior of Endoleaks and Endotension

1. *If a type I or type III endoleak is detected and then sealed [cannot be visualized on computerized tomographic (CT) scans], it will have no bad consequence.*

Of the 26 respondents, 20 disagreed, although one stated that it could happen, and another indicated that it could if abdominal aortic aneurysm (AAA) shrinkage occurred. Thus, consensus was reached that type I and type III endoleaks will have serious consequences even if sealing appears to have occurred. The implication is that pressure can be transmitted through clot.

2. *If a type II endoleak is detected and then sealed (cannot be visualized on CT scans), it will usually have no bad consequences.*

Twenty-one of the 26 respondents agreed with some qualifications. One commented "unless the AAA enlarges." Thus, consensus was reached that sealed type II endoleaks are usually benign. This question without the word "usually" elicited agreement by only 17 participants, indicating that not all type II endoleaks are benign.

3. *Type II endoleaks, if not present at 30 days, will never develop.*

Eighteen of the 26 respondents disagreed. Thus, consensus was reached that late type II endoleaks could occur.

Consensus Relating to Incidence of Endoleaks and Endotension

4. *What is the total percentage of type I endoleaks at your institution (after 24 hours)?*

The answers ranged from 0 to 30%, with a mean of 7.5%. Twenty of the 26 responses (consensus) ranged from 0 to 10%. One comment indicated that the incidence was dependent on patient selection.

5. *What is the total percentage of type II endoleaks at your institution (after 24 hours)?*

The answers ranged from 5 to 40%, with a mean of 17%. Eighteen of the 26 responses (consensus) ranged from 10 to 25%.

6. *What percentage of type II endoleaks seal and have no detrimental effect?*

The answers ranged from 13 to 100%, with a mean of 53%. Eighteen of the 26 responses (consensus) ranged from 30 to 90%. One comment indicated that most type II endoleaks that seal are those detected at the original procedure. Thus, there was again consensus that most but not all type II endoleaks will seal and behave benignly.

7. *What percentage of patients in your institution will develop delayed endoleaks within 3 years of EVAR?*

Answers ranged from 0 to 30%, with a mean of 10%. Eighteen of the 26 responses (consensus) ranged from 4 to 30%. Although 2 respondents answered 0%, another commented that a delayed endoleak indicated a "missed" endoleak or device failure. However, the consensus was that delayed endoleaks do occur.

*Consensus Relating to Diagnosis of Endoleaks
and Endotension*

> 8. *Contrast CT scans with delayed images are the best method for detecting endoleaks.*

Twenty of the 26 participants agreed. Thus, consensus was reached that CT scans are currently the best method for detecting endoleaks, although comments were made that this method is not sensitive enough and that angiography determines the etiology more specifically.

> 9. *When searching for an endoleak, how long should the delayed views be on the CT scans?*

The responses ranged from 1/2 to 25 minutes, with a mean of 4.1 minutes. Twenty-two of the 26 responses (consensus) ranged from 1 to 5 minutes.

> 10. *Endoleaks can always be detected by appropriately delayed CT scans.*

Twenty-two of the 26 respondents disagreed. Thus, there was consensus that some endoleaks could not be detected by even optimal CT scanning.

> 11. *The etiology of an endoleak can reliably be demonstrated by a CT angiogram.*

Twenty-one of the 26 respondents disagreed. Thus there was consensus that the etiology of an endoleak could not reliably be demonstrated by a CT angiogram.

> 12. *What percentage of endoleaks are detectable on conventional arteriography?*

Answers ranged from 20 to 100%, with a mean of 81%. Most (23/26) respondents (consensus) thought that 50–100% of endoleaks could be detected on conventional arteriography, although several comments indicated that superselective injections and oblique views may be required.

> 13. *Simple diameter measurements are an adequate method to follow AAA size and to document enlargement.*

Eighteen of the 26 respondents agreed. Thus, consensus was reached that simple diameter measurements could document AAA enlargement.

However, comments were made that careful comparative measurements must be made and that focal enlargement could be missed.

14. *Duplex scans are the best method for detecting endoleaks.*

Eighteen of the 26 respondents disagreed. Consensus was, therefore, reached that duplex ultrasonography, although useful, was not the best method for detecting endoleaks. A comment was made that it was not accurate in detecting type II endoleaks.

15. *Current techniques for detecting endoleaks and endotension are adequate.*

Twenty-two of the 26 respondents disagreed. Thus, consensus was reached that current techniques, particularly those for detecting endotension, were inadequate. Several comments indicated that a better method for measuring intrasac pressure is needed.

16. *Better methods are needed to detect endoleaks and endotension.*

Similarly, 24 of 26 respondents (consensus) agreed that better and more sensitive noninvasive methods to detect endoleaks and endotension are needed.

17. *Enlargement of an AAA by more than 0.5 cm is indicative of endotension or an endoleak.*

With some qualifications, 19 of the 26 respondents agreed (consensus). Three believed that an 8 mm size increase is required because of measurement difficulties, and one was more comfortable with volume measurement changes.

Consensus Relating to Prevention and Treatment of Endoleaks and Endotension

18. *Patent lumbar and inferior mesenteric branches should be treated in some way before EVAR.*

Twenty-three respondents disagreed. Thus there was consensus that such pretreatment should not be performed.

19. *Patent hypogastric branches that can reflux into common iliac aneurysms giving rise to endoleaks should be treated in some way prior to EVAR.*

Nineteen of the 26 respondents agreed. Thus, consensus was reached on this issue, although 5 disagreed and 2 were uncertain.

20. *Coils placed within the area of contrast visualization within an excluded AAA sac after EVAR will result in thrombosis of any endoleak and elimination of endotension.*

Twenty-one of the respondents disagreed. Thus, consensus was reached that such sac coiling would be ineffective in treating particularly a type I or type III leak. Even if clot was induced, pressure would be transmitted to the sac wall. A possible exception was thought by some to be a type II leak in which thrombosis of a long branch might lead to decreased sac pressure.

21. *An enlarging AAA after EVAR without evidence of an endoleak should usually be repaired surgically or with a new endograft.*

Twenty of 26 respondents agreed. Thus, consensus was reached on the requirement for aggressive treatment in this circumstance. Two participants expressed the reservation that the AAA must be threateningly large and the patient suitably fit to withstand the procedure.

22. *Occlusion of both hypogastric arteries should never be performed.*

Nineteen of 26 respondents disagreed. Thus, consensus was reached that such bilateral hypogastric interruption may occasionally be necessary and justified, although it was agreed that this should be avoided if possible.

23. *If a type II endoleak is to be repaired, what is your primary method of choice to do so?*

Twenty-two of the 26 respondents indicated that transarterial coil embolization is their preferred method via the hypogastric or superior mesenteric arteries. Several commented that it is essential to get as close to the AAA sac as possible. Several also commented that this method may be ineffective. Two respondents commented that laparoscopic branch clipping (1) was their primary option, although it was the opinion of others that translumbar approaches (2) will gain increasing recognition and utility.

Consensus Relating to AAA Pulsatility and Endoleaks and Endotension

24. *If an AAA is nonpulsatile on physical examination after EVAR, it indicates there is no endoleak or endotension.*

Eighteen of the 26 participants disagreed. Thus, there was consensus that decreased AAA pulsatility on physical examination was not a good method for assuring freedom from an endoleak or endotension. One comment indicated that type II endoleaks rarely cause AAA pulsatility.

C. Near-Consensus or Prevailing Opinion

Near Consensus Relating to Classification of Endoleaks and Endotension and Relationship Between the Two

1. *The current endoleak classification system (types I–IV) is adequate.*

Seventeen of the 26 respondents answered that it is, although with some qualifications. Thus, the prevailing opinion was that, with some modifications, the current classification system for endoleaks and endotension is adequate. The modified classification system is detailed in Table 2. Additional classifiers or descriptors are included in the footnote to Table 2, although the criteria for successful and unsuccessful treatment remain poorly defined.

Finally, endoleaks and endotension may be associated with AAA enlargement, stability, or shrinkage. It was also the prevailing opinion that some endoleaks could not be classified despite all efforts to do so, and that AAA enlargement could sometimes occur in the absence of an endoleak while AAA shrinkage could occasionally occur despite the presence of an endoleak.

2. *The presence of endotension without a visualized endoleak indicates the presence of an endoleak that is sealed (clotted) or otherwise not visualized.*

Sixteen of the 26 respondents agreed. Thus, the prevailing opinion was that endotension indicated the presence of a sealed or clotted endoleak (i.e., a "virtual endoleak"). One comment indicated that pressure can be transmitted through clot, a point on which there was general agreement. Another comment suggested that pressure could be transmitted to the AAA sac through an intact graft, and another comment indicated that infection in the excluded AAA sac could result in endotension without an endoleak.

3. *Type II endoleaks have no correlation with bad outcomes.*

Sixteen of the 26 respondents disagreed. Thus, there was near-consensus (prevailing opinion) that type II endoleaks could in some instances lead to

Table 2. Classification Scheme for Endoleaks and Endotension[a]

Type	Description
Endoleak	
I	Attachment site leaks[b]
A	Proximal
B	Distal
C	Iliac Occluder[c]
II	Branch leaks[d]
A	Simple or to-and-fro (from only 1 patent branch)
B	Complex or flow through (with 2 or more patent branches)
III	Graft defect[b]
A	Midgraft hole
B	Junctional leak or disconnect
C	Other failure mechanisms (suture holes, etc.)
IV	Graft wall porosity
Endotension[e]	
A	With no endoleak
B	With sealed endoleak (virtual endoleak)
C	With type I or type III leak[f]
D	With type II leak[f]

[a] Endoleaks and endotension can also be classified based on the time of first detection as **perioperative**, within 24 hours of EVAR; **early**, 1–90 days after EVAR; and **late**, after 90 days. In addition, they can be described as **primary**, from the time of EVAR; **secondary**, appearing only after *not* being present at the time of EVAR; and **delayed**, occurring after a prior negative CT scan. Endoleaks can also be described as **persistent**, **transient** or **sealed**, **recurrent**, **treated successfully** or **treated unsuccessfully**. Endoleaks and endotension may be associated with AAA **enlargement**, **stability**, or **shrinkage**.
[b] Some type I and type III leaks may also have patent branches opening from the AAA sac and providing outflow for the leak.
[c] With aortoiliac endograft and femorofemoral bypass; type IC could also be classified as a type II.
[d] From lumbar, inferior mesenteric, hypogastric, renal, or other arteries.
[e] Endotension (the **strict** definition) is defined here as increased intrasac pressure after EVAR without a visualized endoleak on delayed contrast CT scans. In the **generic** sense, endotension is any elevation of intrasac pressure and occurs with type I, type III, and most type II leaks and endotension in the strict sense.
[f] Detectable only on opening the aneurysm sac.

AAA enlargement and rupture. However, 4 participants believed that type II endoleaks had no correlation with bad outcomes. The remaining 6 were uncertain. It was also agreed (see consensus item 2) that type II endoleaks that were sealed usually had no bad consequences.

4. *Type II endoleaks after EVAR usually produce systemic pressures within the AAA sac.*

Fourteen of 26 respondents agreed. Thus, prevailing opinion was that type II endoleaks could produce systemic pressures within the AAA sac. However, 10 participants disagreed and 2 were uncertain, indicating some disagreement on this important point.

Near-Consensus Relating to the Behavior of Endoleaks and Endotension

5. *What percentage of type II endoleaks produce bad outcomes?*

Answers ranged from 0 to 50%, with a mean of 16%. Fifteen of 26 respondents (prevailing opinion) believed that 2–15% of type II endoleaks were associated with bad outcomes. However, 2 participants commented that this may be because there is also an unrecognized type I leak.

Near-Consensus Relating to Diagnosis of Endoleaks and Endotension

6. *The etiology of an endoleak can only be determined from conventional arteriography.*

Seventeen of the 26 respondents disagreed. Thus, the prevailing opinion was that the etiology of endoleaks cannot only be determined by arteriography. Comments were made that CT scans were more accurate and that the etiology may be difficult to determine, although arteriography can be accurate in most cases.

7. *Stability or absence of shrinkage in AAA diameter after EVAR is indicative of endotension and/or endoleak.*

Fifteen of the 26 respondents disagreed. Thus, the prevailing opinion was that stability of AAA size does not necessarily indicate the presence of an endoleak or endotension. Comments were that large aneurysms (>6 cm in diameter) may not shrink and that AAA shrinkage may take years and depends on the type of endograft used.

Near-Consensus Relating to Treatment of Endoleaks and Endotension

8. *Type II endoleaks should only be repaired if they are associated with AAA enlargement.*

Fourteen of the 26 respondents agreed. Thus, prevailing opinion existed that type II endoleaks should only be repaired if associated with AAA enlargement. One comment indicated that all nonshrinking AAAs with a type II leak should be treated. Another indicated that all endoleaks present 30 days after EVAR should be treated.

9.   *Sequential sac volume measurements are needed to document AAA growth.*

Fourteen of the 26 respondents disagreed. Thus, there was prevailing opinion that volume measurements are not needed to document AAA growth. However, 9 participants thought such measurements were necessary, and 3 were uncertain. Several comments indicated that volume measurements were cumbersome.

10.   *At this time, a good surgical risk patient (<65 years of age with a large AAA) should not be treated with EVAR.*

Fifteen of the 26 respondents disagreed, although with some qualifications. Thus, there was qualified prevailing opinion that EVAR should be considered and offered to good risk patients with large AAAs. The qualifications were that the patient have favorable anatomy for EVAR and that the patient should be informed about the uncertainties and risks of EVAR and open repair, and then have the option to choose one or another procedure. Five participants agreed that EVAR should not be offered to good-risk young (<65 years old) patients, and 6 participants were uncertain.

Near-Consensus Relating to AAA Pulsatility and Endoleaks and Endotension

11.   *If an AAA is pulsatile after EVAR, it is evidence of an endoleak.*

Fifteen of the 26 respondents disagreed. Nine agreed, and 2 were uncertain. Thus, prevailing opinion existed that pulsatility after EVAR was not evidence of an endoleak. Two comments indicated that such AAA pulsatility after EVAR was worrisome but inconclusive.

12.   *Endotension correlates poorly with pulsatility.*

Fourteen of 26 respondents agreed, although 2 disagreed and 10 were uncertain. Thus, the prevailing opinion was that pulsatility correlated poorly with endotension.

Two additional questions that elicited prevailing opinion answers were modified slightly at the oral conference so that the answers became consensus. The answers to consensus item 2 achieved widespread agreement only when the word "usually" was added. The answers to consensus item 21 achieved widespread agreement only when the words "or with a new endograft" were added.

D. Divided Opinions or Disagreement

1. *What percentage of type I endoleaks seal and have no detrimental effect?*

Answers ranged from 0 to 50%, with a mean of 15.5%. There was clearly a bimodal distribution of answers with 10 participants answering that none sealed, and that immediate treatment was required. Nine others thought that 10–50% could seal, but rarely after 2 weeks. One comment indicated that all sealed type I leaks will recur.

2. *Occlusion of both hypogastric arteries when necessary is a reasonably safe procedure and carries an acceptable risk.*

Twelve of 26 respondents agreed and 9 disagreed, while 5 were uncertain. Thus, there was an obvious difference of opinion on this issue.

3. *If type II endoleaks are to be repaired, what is your secondary method of choice?*

Twelve of 26 respondents answered laparoscopic clipping, 7 indicated translumbar coiling, 4 transarterial coil embolization, and 3 open repair.

4. *If type II endoleaks are to be repaired, what is your tertiary method of choice?*

Ten of 26 respondents answered open repair, 7 indicated laparoscopic clipping, 1 transarterial coil embolization, and 2 translumbar coiling.

REFERENCES

1. Wisselink W, Cuesta MA, Berends PJ, et al. Retroperitoneal endoscopic ligation of lumbar and inferior mesenteric artery as a treatment of persistent endoleak after endovascular aortic aneurysm repair. J Vasc Surg 2000; 31:1240–1244.

2. Baum RA, Carpenter JP, Cope C, et al. Aneurysm sac pressure measurements after endovascular repair of abdominal aortic aneurysms. J Vasc Surg 2001; 33:32–41.

3
Overall Comment from the Consensus Process

Frank J. Veith and Takao Ohki
Montefiore Medical Center–Albert Einstein College of Medicine, New York, New York, U.S.A.

Richard A. Baum
Brigham & Women's Hospital and Harvard Medical School, Boston, Massachusetts, U.S.A.

Endoleaks are a major unsolved problem when aortoiliac aneurysms are repaired by endovascular grafts. Yet the nature and significance of these endoleaks in individual patients remain unclear. Moreover, the definition and consequences of endotension and the exact relationship between endotension and endoleaks continue to be controversial. The present consensus process was designed to clarify the nature and significance of these endoleaks and endotension, to elucidate the relationship between these two complications, and to provide an overview of current knowledge and opinion regarding these two vexing problems that impact on the rapidly advancing field of EVAR. It is recognized that many of the consensus opinions expressed by this process will change as new knowledge accumulates. As one participant (Wolf Stelter) commented, "Truth in science cannot be found by voting for it." Nevertheless, it is likely that the conclusions of this consensus process will provide useful information on the incidence of endoleaks and methods to diagnose and treat them. These conclusions should also be helpful to others in the management of specific patient problems and in pointing the way toward investigations designed to advance knowledge and to clarify uncertainties.

Despite the potential limitations of consensus conclusions, several areas of current agreement deserve emphasis. It now appears likely that in some circumstances elevated pressure can be transmitted through clot (1–4). This explains why coil embolization of a type I or type II endoleak may be ineffective. It also explains why some abdominal aortic aneurysms (AAAs) enlarge even when no endoleak can be detected and why endotension may occur without an endoleak (5). Other as yet unproven mechanisms may contribute to endotension and AAA enlargement in the absence of an endoleak (6).

It is now clear that type II endoleaks, although often benign and associated with AAA stability or shrinkage (4), can lead to AAA enlargement and rupture, and that this can occasionally occur when the leak appears to have been sealed by clot (7–9). It is also becoming increasingly well recognized that type II endoleaks can produce intrasac pressures in the systemic range and that translumbar embolization is a more effective method for diagnosis and treatment (10). However, this remains to be proven, and laparoscopic clipping of branches remains a popular alternative (11).

The consensus process produced general agreement that simple computed tomography (CI) scan diameter measurements were adequate to determine AAA size changes after endovascular abdominal aortic aneurysm repair (EVAR). Volume measurements, although superior and a valuable research tool, were believed to be too cumbersome for general usage. However, several participants commented on difficulties that could occur with making accurate AAA diameter measurements on CT scan and that efforts should be made to avoid these pitfalls when determining diameter changes.

Several past concepts were clarified or corrected by the consensus process. AAA pulsatility after EVAR was agreed to be a poor index of the presence or absence of an endoleak and endotension (6,12). Furthermore, although some in the past have believed that failure of AAA shrinkage or size stability after EVAR was evidence of an endoleak or endotension, the current prevailing opinion was that this was not so, particularly with large AAAs. Moreover, CT scanning was generally agreed to be a better diagnostic modality for endoleak detection than duplex ultrasonography.

General agreement existed on several items, which point the way towards future research requirements. Improved techniques for diagnosing endoleaks and particularly endotension are needed. There is presently no method to measure intrasac pressure noninvasively. It was also agreed that hypogastric arteries or branches should not be allowed to retain open communication with the sac of aortoiliac or iliac aneurysms and that unilateral hypogastric embolization was justified. However, bilateral hypogastric occlusion, although sometimes justified, was believed to be best avoided. It was not certain how often this was justified or what would be the best method to avoid it (hypogastric revascularization or branched endografts).

The modified classification scheme (Table 1) was introduced to permit a more detailed categorization of endoleaks and endotension. The greater detail in this scheme will hopefully facilitate communication between investigators and lead to more accurate analyses of the natural history and the effectiveness of

Table 1. Classification Scheme for Endoleaks and Endotension

Type	Description of source of perigraft flow
Endoleak[a]	
I	Attachment site leaks[b]
A	Proximal end of endograft
B	Distal end of endograft
C	Iliac occluder (plug)
II	Branch leaks[c] (without attachment site connection)
A	Simple or to-and-fro (from only 1 patent branch)
B	Complex or flow through (with 2 or more patent branches)
III	Graft defect[b]
A	Junctional leak or modular disconnect
B	Fabric disruption (midgraft hole)
	(i) Minor(<2 mm) e.g., suture holes
	(ii) Major (≥ 2 mm)
IV	Graft wall (fabric) porosity (<30 days after graft placement)
Endotension[d]	
A	With no endoleak
B	With sealed endoleak (virtual endoleak)
C	With type I or type III leak[e]
D	With type II leak[e]

[a] Endoleaks can also be classified based on the time of first detection as **perioperative**, within 24 hours of EVAR; **early**, 1–90 days after EVAR; and **late**, after 90 days. In addition, they can be described as **primary**, from the time of EVAR; **secondary**, appearing only after *not* being present at the time of EVAR; and **delayed**, occurring after a prior negative CT scan. Endoleaks can also be described as **persistent, transient,** or **sealed, recurrent, treated successfully** or **treated unsuccessfully.** Endoleaks and endotension may be associated with AAA **enlargement, stability** or **shrinkage.**
[b] Some type I and type III leaks may also have patent branches opening from the AAA sac and providing outflow for the leak.
[c] From lumbar, inferior mesenteric, hypogastric, renal, or other arteries.
[d] Endotension (the **strict** definition) is defined here as increased intrasac pressure after EVAR without a visualized endoleak on delayed contrast CT scans. In the **generic** sense, endotension is any elevation of intrasac pressure and occurs with type I, type III and most type II leaks and endotension in the strict sense.
[e] Detectable only on opening the aneurysm sac.

treatment methods for the various types and subtypes of endoleaks. These goals also underlie our definition of "endotension." Obviously pressure is elevated within an aneurysm sac after EVAR with all types of endoleaks (endotension in the generic sense). However, the strict usage of the term "endotension" within our classification scheme is reserved for circumstances in which the intrasac pressure is elevated *without a demonstrable endoleak* on a delayed contrast CT scan. This definition and classification scheme will permit a more accurate categorization of the circumstances in individual patients. This in turn will permit more accurate determination of natural history and prognosis and more precise application of the most appropriate treatment.

The classification scheme presented in Table 1 includes a category for endotension without any endoleak (type A) even at open operation, and we and others have described such cases. It also includes a category (type B) with a sealed or clotted endoleak. This would be considered a virtual endoleak because there is no blood flow outside the grafts in the sac. Only when clot is removed from the branch orifice at operation does the leak become apparent and we have had such a case (9). In addition, patients with a type I or type III endoleak may not have it visualized on a CT scan but may still have a high intrasac pressure (type C), and patients with a type II endoleak may not have a leak visualized but still have a high intrasac pressure (type D). In these latter two categories, the endoleak only becomes apparent when the aneurysm sac is opened at operation. Whether patients with type C and type D behave like those with type I and III leaks and type II leaks, respectively, remains to be determined.

In conclusion, the consensus process achieved remarkable agreement among leaders in the field from many countries. This agreement should be helpful in guiding current patient management. In addition to reaching consensus or near-consensus on a number of complex and controversial issues, all the participants agreed that much remained to be learned about endoleaks and endotension and how they may be prevented and treated. These perplexing problems will continue to be a challenge to the success of EVAR and will have to be addressed aggressively by those interested in the field. Until solutions to these problems are found, EVAR will remain an imperfect long-term treatment and continued periodic follow-up to detect and treat them will be mandatory.

REFERENCES

1. Marty B, Sanchez LA, Ohki T, et al. Endoleak after endovascular graft repair of experimental aortic aneurysms: does coil embolization with angiographic "seal" lower intraaneurysmal pressure? J Vasc Surg 1998; 27(3):454–462.

2. Fisher RK, Brennan JA, Gilling-Smith GL, et al. Continued sac expansion in the absence of demonstrable endoleak is an indication for secondary intervention. Eur J Vasc Endovasc Surg 2000; 20:96–98.

3. Mehta M, Ohki T, Veith FJ, et al. All sealed endoleaks are not the same: a treatment strategy based on an ex vivo analysis. Eur J Vasc Endovasc Surg 2001; 21(6):541–544.

4. Schurink GWH, van Baalen JM, Viser MJT, et al. Thrombus within an aortic aneurysm does not reduce pressure on the aneurysm wall. J Vasc Surg 2000; 31:501–506.

5. Gilling-Smith G, Brennan J, Harris P, et al. Endotension after endovascular aneurysm repair: definition, classification, and strategies for surveillance and intervention. J Endovasc Surg 1999; 6:305–307.

6. White GH, May J. How should endotension be defined? History of a concept and evolution of a new term. J Endovasc Ther 2000; 7:435–438.

7. Zarins CK, White RA, Fogarty TJ. Aneurysm rupture after endovascular repair using the AneuRx stent graft. J Vasc Surg 2000; 31(5):960–970.

8. Politz JK, Newman VS, Stewart MT. Late abdominal aortic aneurysm rupture after AneuRx repair: a report of three cases. J Vasc Surg 2000; 31:599–606.

9. Sahgal A, Veith FJ, Lipsitz E, et al. Diameter changes in isolated iliac artery aneurysms 1 to 6 years after endovascular graft repair. J Vasc Surg 2001; 33(2):289–295.

10. Baum RA, Carpenter JP, Cope C, et al. Aneurysm sac pressure measurements after endovascular repair of abdominal aortic aneurysms. J. Vasc Surg 2001; 33:32–41.

11. Wisselink W, Cuesta MA, Berends PJ, et al. Retroperitoneal endoscopic ligation of lumbar and inferior mesenteric artery as a treatment of persistent endoleak after endovascular aortic aneurysms repair. J Vasc Surg 2000; 31:1240–1244.

12. Greenberg R, Green R. A clinical perspective on the management of endoleaks after abdominal aortic endovascular aneurysm repair. J Vasc Surg 2000; 31:836–837.

4

Endoleak and Endotension: Definitions, Classification, and Current Concepts

Geoffrey H. White
University of Sydney and Royal Prince Alfred Hospital, Sydney, New South Wales, Australia

I. INTRODUCTION

Development of endoluminal techniques for aneurysm repair has been accompanied by previously unencountered complications. The most interesting and demanding of these are incomplete seal of the endovascular graft ("endoleak") and persistent growth or pressurization of the aneurysm sac without extragraft blood flow ("endotension"). The defining factor for endoleak is thus blood flow, whereas endotension implies growth or pressure without blood flow. Both of these phenomena may be due to misplacement or poor sizing of the endovascular graft device (technical error), may be the result of material fatigue, displacement, or distortion (device failure), or may be precipitated by specific reactions to the graft device within the environment of the aneurysm sac (patient factors). Endoleak has been perceived as the Achilles' heel of endovascular technology—the incidence and severity of this complication and its relationship to long-term procedure outcome will influence to a great degree the eventual acceptance of the endovascular repair technique.

This chapter presents concepts and definitions of endoleak and endotension and they have evolved during the early history of the development of endovascular grafting, with associated discussion of clinical presentation, patient investigation, and basics of management as previously presented in early manuscripts on these subjects. The purpose of the chapter is thus to act as an introduction and general primer for the more detailed work presented elsewhere in this book.

II. ENDOLEAK

A. Definition

Endoleak is now widely accepted as a term to describe "a condition associated with endoluminal vascular grafts defined by the persistence of blood flow outside the lumen of the endoluminal graft but within an aneurysm sac or adjacent vascular segment being treated by the graft" (1,2). The most serious form of endoleak is that due to incomplete sealing or exclusion of the aneurysm sac or vessel segment, as evidenced by imaging studies such as contrast-enhanced computed tomography (CT) scan, ultrasound, or angiography. Endoleak may also be caused by blood entering the aneurysm sac by retrograde flow from patent collateral vessels, particularly the lumbar arteries or inferior mesenteric artery, even when a complete seal has been obtained around the endoluminal graft (2,3). Other forms of endoleak are due to device failure, in particular when associated with modular graft disconnection or with blood flow through tears in the wall of an endovascular graft fabric.

B. Classification

Classification of endoleak is presented in Tables 1 and 2. A distinction is made between endoleak related to incomplete seal around the graft device at the attachment sites (type I) (Fig. 1) and endoleak associated with retrograde flow from collateral arterial branches (type II) (Fig. 2) (4). Two further subgroups of graft-related endoleak are recognized, both describing persistent flow related to the defects in the wall or midgraft region of the endovascular graft or device (5). Thus, endoleak due to fabric tears, graft disconnection, or disintegration is classified as type III (Fig. 3), and flow through the graft presumed to be associated with graft wall "porosity" is termed type IV (Fig. 4) (5).

All subgroups may be further defined as primary (early) or secondary (late), or by site (2).

> Type I Endoleak (perigraft endoleak, graft-related endoleak, or attachment-site endoleak): This occurs when a persistent perigraft channel of blood flow develops due to inadequate or ineffective seal at the graft ends (at the proximal, or distal graft aspects) or "attachment zones."

Table 1. Classification of Endoleak

Time of occurrence
  Primary endoleak: Endoleak present from the time of the implantation procedure or diagnosed during the 30-day perioperative period
  Secondary endoleak (or late endoleak): Endoleak occurring as a late event after successful endoluminal graft implantation procedure
Site
  Graft-related (perigraft endoleak)
    Proximal endoleak (proximal perigraft channel)
    Midgraft endoleak (intersegmental perigraft channel)
    Distal endoleak (distal perigraft channel)
    Graft wall endoleak through fabric
  Non–graft-related (retrograde endoleak)
    Lumbar collateral flow into sac
    Mesenteric collateral flow into sac
    Other collateral branch flow into sac (iliac, intercostal)

Type II Endoleak (retrograde endoleak or non–graft-related endoleak): This occurs when there is persistent collateral blood flow into the aneurysm sac flowing retrogradely from patent lumbar arteries, the inferior mesenteric artery, or other collateral vessels. In this case, there is a complete seal around the graft attachment zones so that the complication is not related directly to the graft itself.

Type III Endoleak (fabric tear or modular disconnection): Endoleak at the midgraft region may be due to leakage through a defect in the graft fabric or between the segments of a modular, multisegment graft. This subgroup of endoleak is essentially due to mechanical failure of the graft, secondary to early component defect or late material fatigue. Some cases may be associated with the effects of hemodynamic forces or changes in aneurysm morphology with shrinkage.

Type IV Endoleak (graft porosity): Any minor blush of contrast on completion angiogram or subsequent contrast studies, which is presumed to be emanating from blood diffusion across the pores of a highly porous graft fabric within the initial few days after graft implantation, or perhaps through the small holes in the graft fabric caused by sutures or stent struts, etc. This is an inherent feature of some graft designs, rather than a form of device failure. In practice, differentiation of type IV endoleak from other types of endoleak is often quite difficult and may require postoperative,

Table 2. Treatment Options for Endoleak and Endotension

Classification	Alternative terms	Forms	Rx alternatives
Type I Endoleak	Attachment endoleak	Proximal graft attachment zone	Proximal or distal extension or cuff
	Perigraft channel Perigraft leak Graft-related endoleak	Distal attachment zone	Embolization Secondary endograft Open repair
Type II Endoleak	Retrograde endoleak Collateral flow Retroleak	Patent lumbar artery Patent IMA Patent intercostal artery	Conservative Coil embolization Laparoscopic clip application
	Non–graft-related endoleak	Others (accessory renal artery, internal iliac, subclavian etc.)	
Type III Endoleak	Fabric tear Modular disconnection or poor seal	Midgraft fabric tear Contralateral stump disconnection	Secondary endograft
Type IV Endoleak	Porosity	Graft wall fabric porosity; suture holes	Conservative
Endoleak of undefined origin			
Endotension	Endopressure Pressure leak Pseudo-endoleak	High pressure in sac, but no endoleak shown Thrombotic seal	Secondary endograft Open repair ?Others

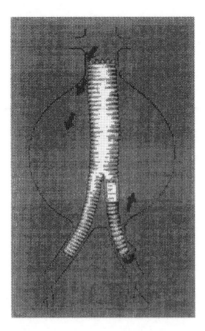

Figure 1. Type I endoleak is defined as incomplete seal of the aneurysm sac at the proximal or distal attachment zones of the endograft device. This may result from endograft undersizing, angulation, or short length of the aneurysm neck, irregular aortic or iliac artery wall, or folds of the device wall resulting in a flow channel into the sac.

        precise ultrasound studies or directed angiography. As yet, the long-term effects of type IV endoleak are unknown, but in some instances late recurrence in the form of "microleaks" has been reported (6).

Endoleak of Undefined Origin: In many cases, the precise source of endoleak will not be clear from routine follow-up imaging studies, and further investigation may be required. In this situation, it may be appropriate to classify the condition as "endoleak of undefined origin" until the type of endoleak is precisely defined by further studies.

For endoleaks of types I–III, further specificity many be gained by adding the qualifiers A or B, where A refers to endoleaks in which only an inflow channel can be imaged and B refers to endoleak with demonstrated inflow and outflow channels (5).

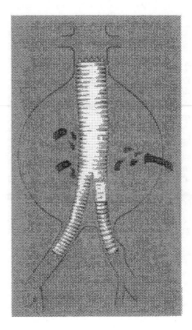

Figure 2. Type II endoleak results from retrograde blood flow from lumbar, mesenteric, or other branch vessels.

Non–endoleak Aneurysm Sac Pressurization (endotension): In these cases, no endoleak is demonstrated on imaging studies, but pressure within the aneurysm sac is elevated and may be very close to systemic pressure (5,7). The seal is formed by semi-liquid thrombus, and the pressure in the sac is similar to pressures measured in endoleak. The aneurysm will often be clinically pulsatile and wall-pulsatility may also be detected and monitored by specialized ultrasound techniques (8).

Precise classification of these various types of endoleak allows more meaningful communication and comparison of results from different investigators and different devices. In addition, treatment recommendations can be made according to the type of endoleak, as well as its site. For example, type III endoleak (fabric tear or modular separation) can be effectively treated in many cases by insertion of a further endograft to line and reinforce the graft wall or connection zone where the defect is detected (9,10), whereas type II

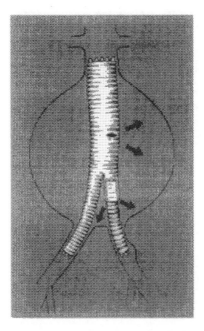

Figure 3. Type III endoleak is defined by blood flow leakage into the sac through a defect of the endograft wall (e.g., fabric tear) or from the overlap zone of two components of a modular graft.

endoleak may be managed quite differently by transluminal coil embolization (11,12). There is good case for conservative management of type II endoleak when there is no aneurysm enlargement; recent evidence demonstrated that there was no significant increase in abdominal aortic aneurysm (AAA) size over 12–18 months in series of patients who had primary type II endoleak (13,14). Follow-up studies for endovascular devices should present differential information for each type of endoleak, so that their incidence, prognosis, and best treatment can ultimately be determined (15).

It is likely that other subgroups of endoleak will be recognized as the design of endovascular grafts evolves and as imaging techniques become more advanced.

C. Timing of Endoleak

Primary endoleak is considered to exist when it is detected during the perioperative (30-day) period. Since flow into the aneurysm sac may also

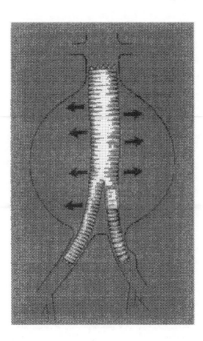

Figure 4. Type IV endoleak represents minor blood leakage into the aneurysm sac due to inherent porosity of the device fabric. This appears as a blush of contrast on angiographic images; the term is applicable only to blush flow detected on angiogram or early CT imaging during the perioperative interval.

become reestablished as a late complication after apparent initial complete seal, a separate entity should be recognized as secondary endoleak.

Secondary endoleak, (otherwise referred to as "delayed" or "late endoleak," occurs after the perioperative 30-day interval or after there has been an initial sealing of the AAA. This problem is receiving increased attention as one of the major long-term complications of the endoluminal grafting technique (2,16). Late endoleak of type I or type III classification is equivalent to aneurysm recurrence and may be complicated by aortic rupture (17–21). Active intervention (secondary endoluminal graft procedures, percutaneous stenting or embolization procedures, or other interventions) is recommended for all patients who develop late endoleak of type I or type III to prevent AAA rupture.

Type II endoleak seems empirically far less likely to lead to aneurysm rupture, whether it occurs as a primary or a secondary event. There have been no published reports of aortic aneurysm rupture associated with late type II endoleak to date. Nevertheless, it is instructive to consider that rupture has been reported due to backflow from collateral vessels of an AAA treated by surgical ligation and extra-anatomical bypass (22), and occult type II endoleak was considered to be the probable cause of rupture of an internal iliac aneurysm in one reported case (23). Thus, even though the current management of primary or late endoleak of type II origin is usually conservative, many cases of type II endoleak have been treated by percutaneous embolization techniques, especially when they persist longer than 6–12 months or are associated with AAA enlargement.

D. Graft Porosity and Difficulties in Differentiating Source of Endoleak

It is recognized that, with thin-walled graft materials, endoleak in the early few days after endograft procedures may be due to graft porosity or to small holes in the graft wall caused by suture attachment of the metallic stent to the graft and that these "pores" may close spontaneously within a short period. In current experience with the AneuRx graft, for example, a "blush" of contrast is seen within the aneurysm sac on completion angiography in the large majority of cases done, and contrast is demonstrated outside the graft on CT scan done 2–5 days postoperatively in approximately one quarter to one third of cases. Many of these resolve within the first month (24). This suggests that sealing of pores or flow channels has occurred.

Some have taken the viewpoint that such blood flow through the graft wall is insignificant, that it is not a form of endoleak, and that sealing of these holes equates to a successful procedure (24). The corollary of this attitude, which some investigators seem to have adopted, is that all early flow in the sac should therefore be regarded as harmless until it is proven not to be. There are several telling arguments against this attitude: (1) It can be extremely difficult to determine accurately if blush flow outside the graft on completion angiography or on early postoperative CT scan is actually endoleak around the ends, or through a modular connection site, or simple flow through graft pores; (2) it has been shown that endoleak through a hole of any size, even a very small one, results in identical high pressure within the AAA sac (25); (3) pressure in the aneurysm sac remains high after endoluminal repair with a porous graft, in benchtop model studies (25), and (4) the long-term outcome of this phenomenon is unknown, and it is feasible that graft porosity may be found to be associated with late complications such as continued enlargement of the aneurysm sac, recurrent endoleak, etc. Recently a phenomenon of so-called "microleak" has been identified in late follow-up of such cases, characterized by small jets of blood and/or contrast media projecting through the fabric wall on angiographic or ultrasound studies (6).

One aspect that requires clinical investigation is whether pressure reduction within the aneurysm sac is achieved as effectively when the seal of small pores or channels in the graft wall is thrombotic rather than structural; thrombus (or fibrin plug) sealing a flow channel may possibly transmit higher pressures to the interior of the aneurysm sac leading to different pressure effects on the aortic wall in both the early and late stages. In fact, it has been demonstrated in experimental studies that coil embolization of endoleak channels associated with holes in the graft fabric does not effectively reduce sac pressure, even though no endoleak can be demonstrated after the thrombosis has been induced (26). It is feasible, therefore, that there may be differences in pressure transmission through holes or pores of various sizes, which have been sealed by thrombus of varying composition, and that these differences may lead to a differential tendency for the thrombosed aneurysm sac to shrink or perhaps to enlarge. Benchtop studies of thrombosed endoleak channels within branch vessels showed that sealing by thrombus does not prevent pressure transmission, but that there is a reduction in pressure which is directly proportional to the length of the endoleak channel and inversely proportional to its diameter (27).

E. Etiology and Incidence

Factors that may play a role in the etiology of endoleak are presented in Table 3. There has been wide variation in the incidence of endoleak reported in series to date. Moore and Rutherford reported a primary endoleak rate of 44% for the initial multicenter trial of the EVT device (28), with more than half of these cases being short-term, self-sealing endoleak, leaving a persistent primary endoleak rate of 21%. Marin et al. reported primary endoleak in 27% of cases (29), including some that progressed to spontaneous thrombosis. Blum et al. (4%) (30), May et al. (9%) (31), and Parodi (32) all reported an incidence of 10% or less. The incidence of primary endoleak probably depends on the device being used, patient anatomical features, the experience of the operative team in patient selection and implantation techniques, and other factors (see Table 3).

In most series the incidence of secondary endoleak increases gradually with longer follow-up and may often be associated with degenerative changes in the graft structure or fabric integrity over time, particularly beyond the initial 2–3 years. Recent reports have shown that some types of endovascular graft devices tend to buckle or kink due to changes in the morphology of the

Table 3.   Etiology of Endoleak

Graft-related factors
  Problems in graft sizing or patient selection
    Graft size mismatch (length/diameter)
    Graft overlap zone mismatch (length/diameter)
    Mismatch of graft shape to aortic morphology (e.g., rigid stent in angulated
      aneurysm neck)
  Unfavorable aortic morphology
    Short neck or attachment zone
    Angulated neck or irregular lumen shape
    Thrombus in neck
  Graft damage
    Graft tear/fragile graft fabric
    Graft tear/suture damage to graft fabric
    Graft perforation due to guidewire perforation
    Graft dilatation
    Balloon or sheath trauma to graft
    Late graft distortion, disconnection, or failure
  Implantation technique problems
    Graft misplacement
    Graft displacement
    Incomplete graft expansion
Non–graft-related factors
    Large patent lumbar arteries
    Large patent inferior mesenteric artery
    Large patent intercostal arteries (thoracic endograft)
    Other collateral flow

excluded aneurysm or due to the relentless hemodynamic stresses placed upon the device (33,34). Grafts that have undergone these structural changes showed a higher incidence of late endoleak and device failure (33,34). Closely monitored prospective studies of long-term outcome will be required before the durability of endoluminal repair and best choice of devices can be defined.

F. Severity

The severity of endoleak probably depends on the size of the perigraft channel and the flow within it, so that small endoleaks may have less tendency to cause major complications. It has been shown that endoleak may seal in the early postoperative stage or at a later time, presumably by a process of thrombosis.

The long-term outcome of sealed endoleak is undefined but it is known that recurrence of endoleak after initial spontaneous sealing is relatively common and that rupture may result. With further experience it may become possible to further define degrees of endoleak as minor (i.e., likely to seal safely by thrombotic process) or major (unlikely to seal or sealed by unstable thrombus with maintained high pressure within the aneurysm sac or high potential for recurrence). Aneurysm rupture has been reported in patients with persistent major endoleak (17–20). Pressure monitoring may be shown to have a valuable role in determining the severity and long-term behavior of different degrees and types of endoleak.

Some have taken the viewpoint that a large caliber patent inferior mesenteric artery or large lumbars (particularly the fourth lumbar arteries) should be embolized preoperatively or intraoperatively. Although the prognosis of this type II endoleak appears to be relatively favorable during the first 12–18 months (3,13,14), it is also possible that longer-term persistent retrograde perfusion of the aneurysm sac may go on to cause secondary changes to the biological reactions within the aneurysm thrombus, to the geometry of the aneurysm sac, or to the graft wall, any of which could result in late deleterious alterations in graft geometry or integrity.

G. Management

Management of endoleak may be considered under five broad categories:

1. Conservative: observation, with monitoring by repeat imaging
2. Embolization: percutaneous embolization, by trans-arterial route or by direct trans-lumbar
3. Secondary endograft: correction by further endoluminal graft procedure
4. Surgical modification: transabdominal or laparoscopic band-ligature of the aortic neck
5. Conversion: to open repair of aneurysm

We have previously emphasized the possibility of aneurysm rupture in patients with late endoleak where conservative management had been preferred to active intervention (19). Seven of 8 patients who suffered this complication as a late event survived emergency open repair of the ruptured aneurysm. On the other hand, in our experience only one patient with primary type I endoleak has suffered aneurysm rupture in the early postoperative period, although most patients have undergone early active intervention to correct the endoleak.

The appropriate management depends on the severity of endoleak, the timing of detection, and medical status of the patient. Endoleak detected during the implant procedure on completion arteriogram can often be corrected by balloon dilatation of unexpanded graft segments or by further endograft cuffs or extensions.

Percutaneous embolization is reserved mostly for closure of type II endoleaks when the aneurysm is symptomatic or enlarging. Embolization with coils or other materials has proven unsatisfactory management for type I or III endoleak, according to anecdotal reports. Thrombosis of the endoleak channel may be achieved, but pressures tend to remain high and recurrent endoleak is common.

It may be possible to close endoleak by placement of a further endoluminal graft, cuff, or coated stent. It is essential to have available a "toolbox" containing a variety of such devices to enable immediate correction of endoleak or graft misplacement. Such adjunctive or secondary procedures are of great value in the management of primary or late endoleak of type I or type III.

Open repair of the aneurysm may be required in some cases where the morphology of the aorta or the graft problem causing endoleak cannot be safely managed by endovascular techniques or when attempts at secondary endovascular repair are unsuccessful (35). If a patient is in an extremely high-risk group, it may be determined that it is safer to manage the case conservatively than to resort to open repair.

III. ENDOTENSION

In clinical practice it is now appreciated that high pressure may be maintained within the AAA sac with no evidence of "leak" or bloodflow outside the graft, particularly in cases where a rim of thrombus is interposed between the sac contents and the aortic lumen (7), but also as a consequence of other mechanisms. Early observations of this phenomenon were associated with distal displacement or slip of the upper aspect of devices from within the proximal aneurysm neck; the aneurysm became pulsatile once more and was enlarging on progress CT scans, but no contrast media was detected outside of the graft (7). In other circumstances, the abdominal aortic aneurysm may continue to expand following apparently successful repair by endoluminal graft technique, with no evidence of endoleak on imaging studies, no evidence of stent displacement, and a nonpulsatile AAA sac on clinical examination. It has been theorized that this phenomenon is due in most cases to maintenance of high pressure within the aneurysm sac, presumably by pressure transmission from the adjacent aortic lumen (5,7). A likely mechanism in many such cases is transmission of a damped pressure wave through thrombus which is acting to seal the endograft from flowing blood, but which is not an adequate barrier to totally exclude the aneurysm sac from pressure effects. In other cases, endoleak may be present but not detected due to inadequately performed imaging or a low flow rate.

Whenever an aneurysm is noted to increase in size [maximal diameter, or volume (36)], the question must arise as to whether endoleak is present. Endoleak may be missed on CT scan if the images are obtained early in the cycle after infusion of the vascular contrast medium; late CT images should also be obtained to demonstrate retrograde flow from collateral arteries, or delayed blood flow in the AAA sac occurring through the graft wall (type III) or through small channels around the ends of the graft (type I). If no endoleak is detected on any imaging studies, then endotension is suspected.

In two cases of endotension treated by late conversion to open repair, we were able to obtain measurements of intrasac pressures; the systolic pressures within the thrombus were similar to systemic pressures (7), and the operative findings supported the theory that this was due to high pressures within the aneurysm sac being transmitted through a layer of thrombus or semi-liquid thrombotic gel, leading to continued expansion of the AAA.

Several groups have measured pressures within the aneurysm through a catheter adjacent to the endovascular graft (25,37,38). Chuter et al. (37) demonstrated that exclusion of an aneurysm by endovascular graft leads to a significant reduction of intrasac pressures; mean aneurysm pressure was 36.5/33.8 mmHg compared to mean radial arterial pressures of 118.5/50.5. These findings corresponded with a reduction in the palpable pulse and an absence of perigraft flow on follow-up CT scans. On the other hand, Stelter and coworkers showed that intra-aneurysmal pressures remained high when endoleak channels occurred, using a similar methodology (38). Noninvasive methods of measuring intra-aneurysmal pressures are not yet available; Malina et al. suggested that an indirect indication may be obtained from ultrasound monitoring of aortic wall pulsatility (8). Implantable pressure transducers may give valuable evidence regarding pressure profiles in patients with and without endoleak in future studies, thus adding to the current knowledge of endotension.

Alternative mechanisms leading to continued aneurysm growth despite evidence of radiographic exclusion have not been fully elucidated (39). It is logical to assume that a contributing factor in many cases is transmission or maintenance of systemic blood pressure within the sac. However, an increase in sac volume cannot occur without accumulation of more luminal content.

Ongoing thrombus accumulation suggests circulatory inflow, but no outflow. "Endotension" may represent a form of endoleak so slow that blood clots at the source of leakage. Ongoing degradative processes in the arterial wall may be an additional mechanism of sac growth by wall thinning.

Deployment of an endograft low in the aortic neck or later displacement of the proximal attachment segment may be causative factors for endotension due to pressure transmission through a lining or rim or thrombus and may represent an intermediate stage in the development of attachment site endoleak. Experience to date would suggest that the presence of high pressure within the AAA sac without endoleak is relatively uncommon but that the incidence may be device-dependent. In our series, endotension was detected in only 4 of the initial 300 patients treated by endovascular grafts, whereas AAA growth without endoleak has been encountered more frequently in later experience with thinner fabric devices.

A. Definition of Endotension

The term "endotension" has been applied to the condition of persistent or recurrent pressurization of the aneurysm sac (7,40). We have proposed the application of the following definition (41): "Endotension is a condition associated with endoluminal vascular grafts, defined by persistent or recurrent pressurization of an aneurysm sac after endovascular repair, without evidence of endoleak. Endotension may be presumed when there is continued growth of the aneurysm sac on progressive imaging studies, and may be proven by pressure measurements or other evidence of stress on the aneurysm wall."

B. Evolution of the Concept of Endotension

The requirement for a new term arose when it was appreciated that aneurysms treated by endovascular grafts may continue to expand, despite having no evidence of endoleak on follow-up imaging studies. We reported this phenomenon in 3 patients in 1995 (42), and many other trials with various devices have also shown similar findings. Concern was raised at an early stage that spontaneous closure or thrombosis of an endoleak channel may, despite satisfactory CT scan or ultrasound appearance, nevertheless continue to transmit high pressures via the intrasac thrombus (43) and therefore may not protect the patient from aneurysm rupture (42,44). The somewhat unexpected finding of AAA growth after apparent complete exclusion was termed "nonendoleak pressurization of the AAA sac" (5), or "endopressure" (5) when initially discussed at various conferences 2–3 years ago and in related anecdotal reports. Parodi also referred to this finding as "pressure-leak" to differentiate it from endoleak (5). Each of these terms sounded somewhat clumsy, and there was obvious appeal for the more descriptive word "endotension," which was suggested by Gilling-Smith (40) [Gilling-Smith and colleagues proposed an alternative definition for endotension which included high pressure in the aneurysm sac due to endoleak. We believe that the new term "endotension" is a good one, but that the definition should be confined to evidence of persistent or recurrent pressurization of an aneurysm sac after endovascular graft implantation, *without evidence of endoleak* (7).]

Implantable sensors that can transmit intra-aneurysmal pressure are being developed, but currently we are unable to obtain sequential pressure measurements within the sac except by highly invasive means, which makes it difficult to consistently apply a definition of endotension in a truly scientific way. Endotension must often be inferred from growth of the sac over time intervals of 6 months or so; if the aneurysm remains pulsatile to physical examination, there is supportive clinical evidence for the presence of high pressure within the sac. These factors determine that the term will often be applied in a speculative manner (or retrospectively after interventions during which pressure within the sac is monitored, such as conversion to open repair).

There are other difficulties in consistent use of the term endotension, since it is not known whether high pressure is the only mechanism of continued AAA growth. It is quite possible that this may occur under the influence of genetic factors or by a gradual process of accumulation of material within the AAA sac, similar to formation of a seroma around prosthetic grafts used for hemodialysis or arterial bypass. Nevertheless, the term remains satisfactory since "tension" has several alternative interpretations in the mechanical or physical sense, commonly referring to pressure within a fluid, but also being defined as "the action of being stretched or strained" (*Oxford Dictionary*) or "the physical state in which a body is stretched or increased in size" (*Macquarie Dictionary*). Thus, growth of the aneurysm is nicely covered by the term, even in the absence of high pressures.

Pressure in an aneurysm sac is reduced markedly when complete seal is obtained by an endograft (25,37). If endoleak is present, the sac remains pressurized (27,38). The pressure locally within the sac will be equivalent to the blood pressure of the endoleak source, which will usually be equal to systemic pressure unless it comes from an atypical collateral source which for some reason has reduced or damped pressure transmission (27). Pressure profiles within the sac may vary, however, according to the efficiency of seal/exclusion, the size of the endoleak channel, and other factors. The distribution of pressure throughout the sac and its transmission to the aneurysm wall may be influenced to a greater or lesser extent by the distribution of solid thrombus within the sac, the morphological features of the aneurysm, or variations in the transmission of pressure to the aneurysm sac by graft wall movements or oscillations (8), by porous graft materials (25), or by pressure transmission through semi-liquid thrombus which is sealing the graft (7). The ex vivo and animal experiments carried out by Schurink and coworkers have shown that the pressure within an aneurysm is independent of the size of the endoleak (45), but that thrombosis of endoleak channels results in variations of pressure at different sites within the thrombus (46).

These factors might explain why aneurysm size changes can vary in different patients with endoleak; some aneurysms continue to enlarge, while others remain static or even decrease in size. If the endoleak is of type II, then static or decreasing size is more likely than with other types of endoleak (13), although significant enlargement of the sac may still occur (47). Nevertheless, measurement of the pressures within type II endoleaks during retrograde embolization procedures have shown high readings equivalent or close to systemic pressure (48). Thus we must conclude that pressure transmission from type II endoleak may have less effect on AAA growth due to low flow or may tend to be localized or compartmentalized more easily than with direct forms of endoleak, leading to less risk of severe effects such as AAA enlargement, rupture, etc.

Elevated intrasac pressure associated with endotension may be more insidious than endoleak and may be a cause of aneurysm rupture, despite the absence of flow abnormalities detected on monitoring studies (44). Noninvasive methods of pressure measurement within the AAA sac are required to enable postprocedural detection of elevated sac pressures in patients treated with endovascular grafts. The term endotension also conveys the possibility of causes other than pressure applying stress to the aneurysm wall.

IV. CONCLUSIONS

Endoleak and endotension are unusual complications, not previously encountered before the advent of endovascular techniques of aneurysm repair. Their existence results from the fact that the aneurysm sac is not opened, modified, or removed during endoluminal graft implantation. Precise definition of causes and outcomes will be required to determine the best management protocols. There is much scope for basic science and clinical research to elucidate the characteristics of each type of endoleak and the pressure profiles and natural history associated with both endoleak and endotension.

REFERENCES

1. White GH, Yu W, May J. "Endoleak"—A proposed new terminology to describe incomplete aneurysm exclusion by an endoluminal graft (letter). J Endovasc Surg 1996; 3:124–125.

2. White GH, Yu W, May J, Chaufour X, Stephen MS. Endoleak as a complication of endoluminal grafting of abdominal aortic aneurysms: classification, incidence, diagnosis and management. J Endovasc Surg 1997; 4:152–168.

3. Malina M, Ivancev K, Chuter TAM, et al. Changing aneurysmal morphology after endovascular grafting: Relation to leakage or persistent perfusion. J Endovasc Surg 1997; 4:23–30.

4. White GH, May J, Waugh RC, Yu W. Type I and type II endoleaks: a more useful classification for reporting results of endoluminal AAA repair. J Endovasc Surg 1998; 5:189–191.

5. White GH, May J, Petrasek P, Waugh RC, Yu W. Type III and type IV endoleak: toward a complete definition of blood flow in the sac after endoluminal repair of AAA. J Endovasc Surg 1998; 5:305–309.

6. Matsumura JS, Ryu RK, Ouriel K. Identification and implications of transgraft microleaks after endovascular repair of aortic aneurysms. J Vasc Surg 2001; 34:190–197.

7. White GH, May J, Waugh RC, Stephen MS, Harris JP. Endotension: an explanation for continued AAA growth after successful endoluminal repair. J Endovasc Surg 1999; 6:308–315.

8. Malina M, Lanne T, Ivancev K, Lindblad B, Brunkwall J. Reduced pulsatile wall motion of abdominal aortic aneurysms after endovascular repair. J Vasc Surg 1998; 27:624–631.

9. Maleux G, Rousseau H, Otal P, Colombier D, Glock Y, Joffre F. Modular component separation and reperfusion of abdominal aortic aneurysm sac after endovascular repair of the abdominal aortic aneurysm. J Vasc Surg 1998; 28:349–352.

10. Görich J, Rilinger N, Soldner J, Kramer S, Orend KH, Schutz A, Sokiranski R, Bartel M, Sunder-Plassmann L, Scharrer-Pamler R. Endovascular repair of aortic aneurysms: treatment of complications. J Endovasc Surg 1999; 6:136–146.

11. Kato N, Semba CP, Dake MD. Embolization of perigraft leaks after endovascular stent-graft treatment of aortic aneurysms. J Vasc Intervent Radiol 1996; 7:805–811.

12. Van Schie G, Sieunarine K, Holt M, Lawrence-Brown M, Hartley D, Goodman M, Prendergast FJ, Khangure M. Successful embolization of persistent endoleak from a patent inferior mesenteric artery. J Endovasc Surg 1997; 4:312–315.

13. Resch T, Ivancev K, Lindh M, Nyman U, Brunkwall J, Malina M, Lindblad B. Persistent collateral perfusion of abdominal aortic aneurysm after endovascular repair does not lead to progressive change in aneurysm diameter. J Vasc Surg 1998; 28:242–249.

14. Arko FR, Rubin GD, Johnson BL, et al. Type-II endoleaks following endovascular AAA repair: preoperative predictors and long-term effects. J Endovasc Ther 2001; 29:292–308.
15. Chaikof EL, Blankensteijn JD, Harris PL, White GH, Zarins CK, Bernard VM, Matsumura JS, May J, Veith FJ, Fillinger MF, Rutherford RB, Kent KC. Reporting standards for endovascular aortic aneurysm repair. J Vasc Surg 2002; 35:1048–1060.
16. Raithel D, Heilberger P, Ritter W, Schunn C. Secondary endoleaks after endovascular aortic reconstruction. J Endovasc Surg 1998; 5:I-26–I-27.
17. Parodi JC. Endovascular repair of abdominal aortic aneurysms and other arterial lesions. J Vasc Surg 1995; 21:549–555.
18. Lumsden AB, Allen RC, Chaikof EL, et al. Delayed rupture of aortic aneurysms following endovascular stent grafting. Am J Surg 1995; 170:174–178.
19. White GH, Yu W, May J, Waugh RC, Chaufour X, Harris JP, Stephen MS. Three-year experience with the White-Yu endovascular GAD graft for transluminal repair of aortic and iliac aneurysms. J Endovasc Surg 1997; 4:124–136.
20. Torsello GB, Klenk E, Kasprzak B, Umsheid T. Rupture of abdominal aortic aneurysm previously treated by endovascular stentgraft. J Vasc Surg 1998; 28:184–187.
21. Alimi YS, Chakfe N, Rivoal E, et al. Rupture of an abdominal aortic aneurysm after endovascular graft placement and aneurysm size reduction. J Vasc Surg 1998; 28:178–183.
22. Resnikoff M, Darling C, Chang BB, Lloyd WE, Paty PSK, Leather RP, Shah DM. Fate of the excluded abdominal aortic aneurysm sac: longterm follow up of 831 patients. J Vasc Surg 1996; 24:851–855.
23. Bade MA, Ohki T, Cynamon J, Veith FJ. Hypogastric artery aneurysm rupture after endovasculargraft exclusion with shrinkage of the aneurysm: significance of endotension from a "virtual" or thrombosed type II endoleak. J Vasc Surg 2001; 33:1271–1274.
24. Zarins CK, White RA, Schwarten D, et al. AneuRx stent graft versus open surgical repair of abdominal aortic aneurysms: multicenter prospective clinical trial. J Vasc Surg 1999; 29:292–308.
25. Sanchez LA, Faries PL, Marin ML, Ohki T, Parsons RE, Marty B, et al. Chronic intraaneurysmal pressure measurement: an experimental method for evaluating the effectiveness of endovascular aneurysm exclusion. J Vasc Surg 1997; 26:222–230.
26. Marty B, Sanchez LA, Ohki T, Wain RA, Faries PL, Cynamon J, Marin ML, Veith FJ. Endoleak after endovascular graft repair of experimental aortic aneurysms: Does coil embolization with angiographic "seal" lower intraaneurysmal pressure? J Vasc Surg 1998; 27:454–462.
27. Mehta M, Ohki T, Veith FJ, Lipsitz EC. All sealed endoleaks are not the same: a treatment strategy based on an ex-vivo analysis. Eur J Vasc Endovasc Surg 2001; 21:541–544.

28. Moore WS, Rutherford R. Transfemoral endovascular repair of abdominal aortic aneurysm: results of the North American EVT phase 1 trial. J Vasc Surg 1996; 23:543–553.

29. Marin ML, Veith F, Cynamon J, et al. Initial experience with transluminally placed endovascular grafts for the treatment of complex vascular lesions. Ann Surg 1995; 22:449–465.

30. Blum U, Langer M, Spillner G, et al. Abdominal aortic aneurysms: Preliminary technical and clinical results with transfemoral placement of endovascular self-expanding stent-grafts. Radiology 1996; 198:25–31.

31. May J, White GH, Yu W, et al. Surgical management of complications following endoluminal grafting of abdominal aortic aneuryms. Eur J Vasc Endovasc Surg 1995; 10:51–59.

32. Parodi, JC. Endovascular repair of abdominal aortic aneuryms. In: Advances in Vascular Surgery. St. Louis: Mosby-Year Book, 1993:85–106.

33. Harris P, Brennan J, Martin J, Gould D, Bakran A, Gilling-Smith G, Buth J, Gevers E, White D. Longitudinal aneurysm shrinkage following endovascular aortic aneurysm repair is a source of intermediate and late complications. J Endovasc Surg 1999; 6:11–16.

34. Umschied T, Stelter WJ. Time related alterations of shape, position and structure of self-expanding modular aortic stent grafts: a four year single center follow-up. J Endovasc Surg 1999; 6:17–32.

35. May J, White GH, Yu W, et al. Conversion from endoluminal to open repair of abdominal aortic aneurysms: a hazardous procedure. Eur J Vasc Endovasc Surg 1997; 14:4–11.

36. Singh-Ranger R, McArthur T, Raphael M, Lees W, Adiseshiah M. What happens to abdominal aortic aneurysms after endovascular grafting? A volumetric study using spiral CT angiography. J Intervent Radiol 1998; 13:145–146.

37. Chuter T, Ivancev K, Malina M, Resch T, Brunkwall J, Lindblad B, Risberg B. Aneurysm pressure following aneurysm exclusion. Eur J Vasc Endovasc Surg 1997; 13:85–87.

38. Stelter W, Umscheid T, Ziegler P. Three-year experience with modular stent-graft devices for endovascular AAA treatment. J Endovasc Surg 1997; 4:362–369.

39. White GH. What are the causes of endotension? J Endovasc Ther 2001; 8:454–456.

40. Gilling-Smith G, Brennan J, Harris PL, Bakran A, Gould D, McWilliams R. Endotension after endovascular aneurysm repair: definition, classification and implications for surveillance and intervention. J Endovasc Surgery 1999; 6:305–307.

41. White GH, May J. How should endotension be defined? History of a concept and evolution of a new term. J Endovasc Ther 2000; 7:435–438.

42. May J, White GH, Yu W, Waugh RC, Stephen MS, Harris JP. A prospective study of changes in morphology and dimensions of abdominal aortic aneurysms

following endoluminal repair: a preliminary report. J Endovasc Surg 1995; 2:343–347.

43. Schurink GWH, van Baalen JM, Visser MJT, van Bockel JH. Thrombus within an aortic aneurysm does not reduce pressure on the aneurysm wall. J Vasc Surg 2000; 31:501–506.

44. Politz JJ, Newman VS, Stewart MT. Late abdominal aortic aneurysm rupture after AneuRx repair: a report of three cases. J Vasc Surg 2000; 31:599–606.

45. Schurink GWH, Aarts NJM, Wilde J, van Baalen JM, Chuter TAM, Schultz Kool LJ, van Bockel JH. Endoleakage after stent-graft treatment of abdominal aneurysm: implications on pressure and imaging. An in-vitro study. J Vasc Surg 1998; 28:234–241.

46. Schurink GW, Aarts NJ, Van Baalen JM, Kool LJ, Van Bockel JH. Experimental study of the influence of endoleak size on pressure in the aneurysm sac and the consequences of thrombosis. Br J Surg 2000; 87:71–78.

47. Schurink GWH, Aarts NJM, van Baalen JM, Chuter TAM, Schultz Kool LJ, van Bockel JH. Endoleakage after stent-graft treatment of abdominal aneurysm: implications on pressure and imaging. An in-vitro study. Eur J Vasc Endovasc Surg 1999; 17:448–450.

48. Velazquez OC, Baum RA, Carpenter JP, Golden MA, Cohn M, Pyeron A, Barker CF, Criado FJ, Fairman RM. Relationship between preoperative patency of the inferior mesenteric artery and subsequent occurrence of type II endoleak in patients undergoing endovascular repair of abdominal aortic aneurysms: relationship to type II endoleak. J Vasc Surg 2000; 32:777–788.

5

Success of Endovascular Repair of Abdominal Aortic Aneurysms and the Presence of Endoleak: The EUROSTAR Experience

Jacob Buth
Catharina Hospital, Eindhoven, The Netherlands

Peter Lyon Harris
University of Liverpool and Royal Liverpool University Hospital, Liverpool, England

I. INTRODUCTION

The primary indication for endovascular abdominal aortic aneurysm repair (EAR) is to prevent death from aneurysm rupture. Thus, long-term success of the treatment is obtained if the possibility of rupture is eliminated. However, rupture after endograft placement appears to occur in at least 1% of the cases annually, as pointed out in a recently published EUROSTAR report (1). EAR has also failed to meet its purpose if conversion to open repair or other secondary procedures are needed (2,3).

The incidence of failure of EAR is related not only to the complexity of aneurysm morphologies treated but also to variables that are currently less well characterized, including endoleaks (4–11). There is an increasing number of reports proposing that the presence of endoleak in fact equals

See Appendix for list of EUROSTAR Collaborative Centers.

failure of treatment. Endoleaks have the potential to increase aneurysmal sac size and intraluminal pressure and possibly lead to late rupture (12–14). In the present chapter we will focus on the relation of endoleak with the primary and secondary rate of success during follow-up in a large collaborative series of patients, data from whom were collated in the EUROSTAR database. The first-month results were not detailed here as they were the subject of a previous report (15).

II. METHODS

Data from 2964 patients who had EAR between July 1994 and January 2000 were assessed. The number of patients that had a recorded follow-up of 1 month or more was 2463, and this cohort formed the basis of this study. Patients were treated in 87 centers from 17 countries. The mean period of follow-up was 15.4 months (range 1–72 months). A total of 7927 postoperative visits was recorded with a mean of 3.2 visits per patient (range 1–9).

Computed tomography (CT) with contrast enhancement of the abdominal blood vessels was the most frequently used method of imaging at follow-up visits (in 94% of patients). However, contrast angiography (CA, in 1% of patients), magnetic resonance angiography (MRA, in 2% of patients), and duplex imaging (DI, in 3% of patients) were used at the discretion of the responsible physicians.

All endoleaks that were identified at one month and thereafter were included in the analysis. Endoleaks at the completion angiography were not considered. Endoleaks were classified according to the proposed scheme by White et al. (8) into the following categories: type I involved endoleaks originating from the attachment site at the proximal infrarenal aortic neck or from the distal site of the endograft at the iliac or aortic bifurcation level; type II involved reperfusion endoleaks from the inferior mesenteric, lumbar, accessory renal, sacral, and hypogastric arteries; type III included endoleaks from the endograft itself, either from fabric holes or from connections between different modules. In cases in which in a patient different types of endoleaks were observed at different follow-up periods, types I and III were considered above type II for the analysis. The interval between the date of operation and the date on which an endoleak was identified for the first time was used for life table analysis of outcome success rates.

Adverse events, recorded during follow-up, included death of the patient, rupture of the aneurysm, and the requirement of a secondary intervention. In patients who underwent multiple procedures, only the most extensive procedure was taken into account according to the following ranking: transabdominal, femorofemoral, and endovascular reintervention. Results are reported as means and ranges or as percentage of patients with discrete variables. Significant differences between study groups were assessed by log rank testing. Primary and secondary outcome success was defined similar to the criteria used by Zarins et al. (16) to allow a comparison with the results of the present study. Primary outcome success was defined as absence of death, no aneurysm rupture, no conversion to open repair, and no secondary intervention. Secondary outcome success was defined as absence of death, no aneurysmal rupture, and no conversion to open repair. In addition, secondary outcome success not incorporating death in the composite endpoint was determined. Life table comparisons of outcome success rates were calculated for different study groups.

III. RESULTS

Of the 2463 patients that constituted the study cohort, 171 had an endoleak at their first month postoperative assessment and 317 patients had a new-onset endoleak, identified at a later date. In total there were 488 (19.8%) patients in which an endoleak was observed at any time after the endograft implantation. Three groups were distinguished: group A, including 191 patients (7.8%) with a type II endoleak; group B, consisting of 297 patients (12%) with type I or III or multiple endoleaks with a combination of different types; and group C, consisting of 1975 patients who never had an endoleak. A new-onset endoleak was observed in 129 patients (67%) in group A, and in 188 (63%) in group B. Preoperative patient characteristics are summarized in Tables 1 and 2.

One hundred and seventy-two patients died during follow-up. There was no statistical difference in survival between the three study groups. However, only 12 (7.0%) of the patients who died had a cause of death related either to the aneurysm or to EAR. Eight of these patients died because of rupture of the aneurysm, two because of infected endografts, one because of endograft thrombosis, and one as a consequence of a complicated conversion to open aneurysm repair.

The cumulative primary outcome success at 2 years was 72.9% in the overall series, 54.7% in group A, 39.7% in group B, and 90.0% in group C ($p = 0.0001$ to 0.0003 for any group comparison) (Fig. 1). Two-year secondary outcome success was 88.0% in all patients, 84.5% in group A, 85.3% in group B, and 89.0% in group C. Only groups B and C differed significantly ($p = 0.04$)

Table 1.   Patient Characteristics and Comorbid Factors in
2463 Patients with EAR

Age, mean years (range)	70.0 (37–92)
Male gender	92.2
ASA physical status classification	
ASA I	8.9
ASA II	37.4
ASA III & IV	54.5
Diabetes	10.3
Smoking	56.6
Hypertension	58.5
Cardiac hx	58.8

Figures represent percent of patients unless indicated otherwise.
EAR: Endovascular abdominal aortic aneurysm repair. ASA:
American Society of Anesthesiologists.

Table 2.   Dimensions and Variables Representing Aneurysm
Morphology at Preoperative Assessment, Device Brands, Device
Configuration, and Adjunct Procedures in 2463 with EAR

Neck diameter (mm)	22.6 (12–40)
AAA diameter (mm)	55.9 (26–150)
Length of aneurysm (mm)	116.0 (30–265)
Device brand (no. of patients)	
Vanguard	823
AneuRx	607
Talent	315
Stentor	267
EVT/Ancure	108
Excluder	104
Zenith	192
Other	42
Configuration of device (no. of patients)	
Bifurcated	2291
Straight	95
Aorto-uni-iliac	77
Adjunct procedures (no. of patients)	779

Figures represent mean values and ranges unless indicated otherwise.

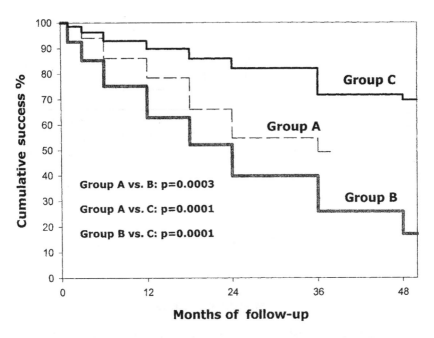

Figure 1.   Primary outcome success rates in groups A, B, and C.

(Fig. 2). If death was not included, the secondary 2-year success rate was 97.4, 88.9, and 98.9% for groups A, B, and C, respectively (Fig. 3). The difference in secondary outcome success omitting death between group A vs. group B and group B vs. group C was significant ($p = 0.006$ and 0.0001, respectively), while there was no difference between groups A and C.

IV. DISCUSSION

Several investigators consider the presence of perigraft flow evidence of failed treatment as it may predict aneurysmal enlargement and eventual rupture (8,17,18). A contrasting opinion was presented in a recent study in which no relationship between the presence of any endoleak and primary and secondary outcome success could be demonstrated (16).

The prevalence of endoleaks during follow-up in the present series was approximately 20%, which is in agreement with persistent endoleak rates observed in other studies (5,19). In 7% of patients endoleaks were present at

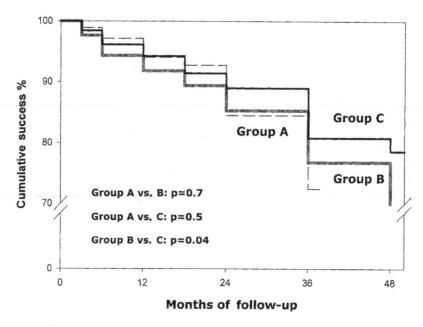

Figure 2. Secondary outcome success rates in groups A, B, and C.

the first month postoperative visit, while in 13% they developed later during follow-up. Matsumura and Moore (5) observed a greater tendency for growth in aneurysms with de novo endoleaks, and these authors suggested that this category may represent a separate entity of endoleaks in which fibrinolysis of initially occluded channels might have taken place. It may be of interest to examine whether a proportion of endoleaks that occur late are in fact initial endoleaks that reappear. This aspect was not investigated here but needs to be addressed in a future study.

Endoleaks originating at the proximal or distal ends of endografts are classified as type I, at the connections of modular prosthesis as type III, and from side branches most commonly lumbar or patent inferior mesenteric arteries as type II (9,20). Occasionally the presence of collateral perfusion is hard to demonstrate. Delayed CT examination with 3 mm slices is probably the best technique to demonstrate collateral reperfusion, and it is definitively better than standard CT (4,21). In this multicenter registry in which CT studies were not uniform, there is a possibility for underdiagnosis of type II endoleak. Contrast-enhanced ultrasound studies may also be more sensitive to small endoleaks (22). Angiography is less sensitive than CT with 3 mm and late

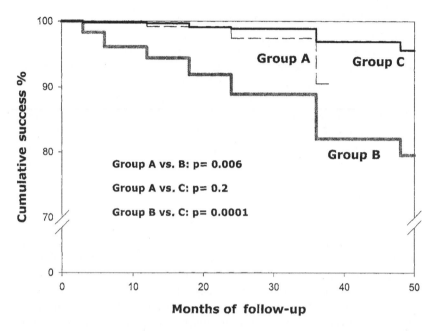

Figure 3. Secondary outcome success, omitting death, from all causes as an adverse event in groups A, B, and C.

films. Not infrequently collateral endoleaks present in combination with endograft related types of endoleaks (1,4). In this study we have separated isolated type II endoleaks from combined endoleaks, which were relegated to group B together with single inflow site device–related endoleaks. Our premise was that collateral endoleaks may follow a course different from graft-related leaks. Moreover, most workers in the field, including ourselves, held the view that the preferred treatment of type II endoleaks is primarily conservative, whereas other endoleaks need a more aggressive approach.

If aneurysms fail to shrink, or even expand, it is assumed they are prone to rupture. From a number of reports it appears that graft-related endoleaks (type I, III, or combinations) are associated with a significantly greater risk of rupture than collateral perfusion (type II) endoleaks (5,23). Others have challenged the concept of a strong correlation between endoleaks and the risk of rupture. In their recent study Zarins and coworkers concluded that some patients who have no endoleaks may decrease their aneurysm and still rupture (16). This led them to conclude that the primary outcome of success, i.e., prevention of rupture, was not necessarily associated with absence of endoleak. In addition, these authors found no difference between primary and secondary rates of success in patients with endoleaks.

Current criteria for success or failure are imperfect. Primary outcome success rate includes the absence of late secondary interventions. It is of note that 76% of late revisions in the EUROSTAR series were by transfemoral technique (2) and may hardly detract from the advantages of EAR. Secondary outcome success takes this consideration into account and combines aneurysm rupture, the occurrence of death from all causes and conversion to open surgery, while omitting other redo procedures. Death during follow-up constitutes another arguable component of outcome success assessment. Late death is infrequently related to the aneurysm or consequences of endovascular repair. In the present study 93% of the late deaths were from causes unrelated to the aneurysm but were due to preexisting conditions or intercurrent diseases typical for this population of patients. Because of this observation we additionally assessed secondary success, omitting death as adverse event. Moreover, to include death in a composite outcome measure will blur the picture if treatment effects in different study groups are compared. Of the deaths related to late rupture, the majority will become apparent after long follow-up periods, given the fact that endovascular-treated AAAs have an annual rupture rate of $1-1\frac{1}{2}\%$ (1). To demonstrate any statistical differences in death rates between distinct patient groups, many years of follow-up are required. These long-term outcomes are not yet available.

In our view the only logical and practical parameters representing secondary outcome success at the current time are rupture of the aneurysm and conversion to open repair. When using these outcome measures, we found significantly worse results in patients with device-related endoleaks compared to patients with collateral endoleaks or no endoleaks at all. Clinical management of endoleaks should be conducted according to these observations.

APPENDIX: PARTICIPANTS OF 87 INSTITUTIONS CONTRIBUTING DATA TO EUROSTAR STUDY

Austria: Vienna—Prof. G. Kretschmer; Belgium: Gilly—Dr. H. Massin; Leuven—Prof. A. Nevelsteen; Bonheiden—Dr. P. M. A. J. Peeters; Turnhout—Dr. P. Stabel; Wilrijk/Antwerp—Dr. M. van Betsbrugge; St. Truiden—Dr. F. van Elst; France: Lyon—Dr. B. Age; Nancy—Dr. C. Amicabile; Paris Creteil cedex—Prof. J. P. Becquemin; Nimes—Dr. Cardon; St. Etienne—Prof. J. P. Favre; Paris cedex—Prof. J. C. Gaux;

Toulouse cedex—Dr. C. Giraud; St. Laurant du Var—Prof. P. Kreitmann; Grenoble—Dr. Magne; Montpellier—Prof. Marty-Ane; Nanterre—Dr. J Marzella; Grenoble cedex—Dr. Meaulle; Draguignan—Dr. C. Mialhe; Marseille—Dr. Piquet; Toulouse—Prof. H. Rousseau; Lille cedex—Dr. M. A. Vasseur; Germany: Mainz—Dr. C. Düber; Düsseldorf—Dr. R. Kolvenbach; Hamburg—Prof. H. Kortmann; Munich—Prof. P. C. Maurer; Ulm—Dr. Pamler; Oldenburg—Dr. Ratusinski; Frankfurt—Prof. W. Stelter; Freiburg—Dr. Uhrmeister; Bonn—Dr. A. Viehofer; Hanover—Dr. G. Voshage; Koblenz—Dr. R. Wickenhoefer; Greece: Psihico Athens—Prof. P. Balas; Ireland: Dublin—Dr. S. Sultan; Israel: Tel Aviv—Prof. B. Morach; Italy: Perugia—Prof. P. Cao; Luxembourg: Luxembourg—Dr. P. Berg; Monaco: Monaco—Dr. C. Mialhe; The Netherlands: Amsterdam—Dr. R. Balm; Nijmegen—Dr. W. B. Barendrecht; Utrecht—Dr. J. Blankensteijn; Eindhoven—Dr. J. Buth; Veldhoven—Dr. J. A. Charbon; Den Haag—Dr. J. C. A. de Mol van Otterloo; Rotterdam—Dr. A. de Smet; Arnhem—Dr. W. R. de Vries; Groningen—Dr. H. R. Dop; Enschede—Dr. R. H. Geelkerken; Tilburg—Dr. L. Hamming; Zwolle—Dr. P. Jörning; Delft—Dr. J. Koning; Tilburg—Dr. S. Kranendonk; Nieuwegein—Dr. F. Moll; Maastricht—Dr. G. W. H. Schurink; Amsterdam—Dr. Vahl; Leiden—Prof. J. H. van Bockel; Rotterdam—Dr. A. C. van der Ham; Den Haag—Dr. H. van Overhagen; Rotterdam—Dr. van Sambeek; Nijmegen—Prof. J van Vliet; Groningen—Dr. E. Verhoeven; Norway: Oslo—Prof. A. Kroeze; Oslo—Prof. K. Kvernebo; Trondheim—Prof. H. Myhre; Poland: Lublin—Prof. Michalak; Spain: Madrid—Dr. E. Criado; Donostia San Sebastian—Dr. M. de Blas; Leon—Dr. R. Fernandez-Samos Gutierrez; Pamplona—Dr. Leopoldo Fernandez Alonso; Lugo—Dr. J. R. Pulpeiro; Barcelona—Dr. V. Riambau; Madrid—Dr. J. A. Sanchez-Corral; Madrid—Dr. D. Stabel; Sweden: Lund—Prof. L. Norgren; Stockholm—Dr. J. Swedenborg; Switzerland: Zurich—Dr. M. Enzler; United Kingdom: Chester—Dr. G. Abbott; Manchester—Dr. R. Asleigh; Bristol—Dr. R. Baird; Bournemouth—Dr. S. Darke; Glasgow—Dr. R. Edwards; Hull—Dr. D. Ettler; Liverpool—Dr. P. Harris; London—Dr. J. Wolfe; New Castle-Upon-Tyne—Dr. M. G. Wyatt.

REFERENCES

1. Harris PL, Vallabhaneni SR, Desgranges P, Becquemin JP, Van Marrewijk C, Laheij RJF. Incidence and risk factors of late rupture, conversion, and death after endovascular repair of infrarenal aortic aneurysms: the EUROSTAR experience. J Vasc Surg 2000; 32:739–749.

2. Lahey RJF, Buth J, Harris PL, Moll FL, Stelter WJ, Verhoeven ELG. Need for secondary interventions after endovascular repair of abdominal aortic aneurysms. Intermediate follow-up results of a European collaborative registry (EURO-STAR). BJS 2000; 87:1666–1673.

3. Cuypers PWM, Laheij RJF, Buth J. Which factors increase the risk of conversion to open surgery following endovascular abdominal aortic aneurysm repair? Eur J Vasc Endovasc Surg 2000; 20:183–189.

4. Resch T, Ivancev K, Lindh M, Nyman U, Brunkwall J, Malina M, et al. Persistent collateral perfusion of abdominal aortic aneurysm after endovascular repair does not lead to progressive change in aneurysm diameter. J Vasc Surg 1998; 28:242–249.

5. Matsumura JS, Moore WS. Clinical consequences of periprosthetic leak after endovascular repair of abdominal aortic aneurysm. J Vasc Surg 1998; 27:606–613.

6. Wain RA, Marin ML, Ohki T, Sanchez LA, Lyon RT, Rozenblit A, et al. Endoleaks after endovascular graft treatment of aortic aneurysms: classification, risk factors, and outcome, J Vasc Surg 1998; 27:69–80.

7. Greenberg R, Green R. A clinical perspective on the management of endoleaks after abdominal aortic endovascular aneurysm repair. J Vasc Surg 2000; 31:836–837.

8. White GH, May J, Waugh RC, Yu W. Type I and type II endoleaks: a more useful classification for reporting results of endoluminal AAA repair. J Endovasc Surg 1998; 5:189–193.

9. White GH, May J, Waugh RC, Chaufour X, Yu W. Type III and type IV endoleak: toward a complete definition of blood flow in the sac after endoluminal AAA repair. J Endovasc Surg 1998; 5:305–309.

10. Gilling Smith G, Brennan J, Harris PL, Bakran A, Gould D, McWilliams R. Endotension after endovascular aneurysm repair: definition, classification, and strategies for surveillance and intervention. J Endovasc Surg 1999; 6:305–307.

11. White GH, May J, Petrasek P, Waugh R, Stephen M, Harris J. Endotension: an explanation for continued AAA growth after successful endoluminal repair. J Endovasc Surg 1999; 6:308–315.

12. May J, White GH, Yu W, Waugh RC, Stephen MS, Harris JP. A prospective study of changes in morphology and dimensions of abdominal aortic aneurysms following endoluminal repair: a preliminary report. J Endovasc Surg 1995; 2:343.

13. Matsumura JS, Pearce PH, McCarthy WJ, Yao JST. Reduction of aortic aneurysm size: early results after endovascular graft placement. J Vasc Surg 1997; 25:113–123.

14. Armon MP, Yusuf SW, Whitaker SC, Gregson RHS, Wenham PW, Hopkinson BR. Thrombus distribution and changes in aneurysm size following endovascular aneurysm repair. Eur J Vasc Endovasc Surg 1998; 16:472–476.

15. Buth J, Laheij RJF. Early complications and endoleaks after endovascular abdominal aortic aneurysm repair: report of a multicenter study. J Vasc Surg 2000; 31:134–146.

16. Zarins CK, White RA, Hodgson KJ, Schwarton D, Fogarty TJ. Endoleak as a predictor of outcome after endovascular aneurysm repair. AneuRx multicenter clinical trial. J Vasc Surg 2000; 32:90–107.
17. Raithel D, Heilberger Ph, Ritter W, Schunn C. Secondary endoleaks after endovascular aortic reconstruction (abstr). J Endovasc Surg 1998; suppl I:I-26–I-27.
18. Sunder-Plassmann L, Orend K, Görich J, Rilinger N, Pamler R. The endoleak issue: main determinant of stent-graft future in endoluminal AAA-repair? (abstr). J Endovasc Surg 1999; 6:208.
19. Broeders IAMJ, Blankensteijn JD, Gvakharia A, May J, Bell PLF, Swedenborg J, et al. The efficacy of transfemoral endovascular aneurysm management: a study on size changes of the abdominal aorta during mid-term follow-up. Eur J Vasc Endovasc Surg 1997; 14:84–90.
20. White GH, Yu W, May J. "Endoleak"—a proposed new terminology to describe incomplete aneurysm exclusion by an endoluminal graft. J Endovasc Surg 1996; 3:124–125.
21. Schurink GWH, Aarts NJM, Wilde J, Van Baalen JM, Chuter TAM, Schultze Kool LJ, et al. Endoleakage after stent-graft treatment of abdominal aneurysm: implications on pressure and imaging—an in vitro study. J Vasc Surg 1998; 28:234–241.
22. Giannoni MF, Bilotta F, Fiorani L, Fiorani P. Reduction in aneurysm size: early results after endovascular graft replacement. J Vasc Surg 1998; 27:981.
23. Malina M, Ivancev K, Chuter TAM, Lindh M, Länne T, Lindblad B, et al. Changing aneurysmal morphology after endovascular grafting: relation to leakage or persistent perfusion. J Endovasc Surg 1997; 4:23–30.

6
Clinical Experience with Endotension: Presentation, Management, and Analysis of Causes

Geoffrey H. White and James May
*University of Sydney and Royal Prince Alfred Hospital, Sydney,
New South Wales, Australia*

An abdominal aortic aneurysm (AAA) may continue to expand following apparently successful repair by endoluminal graft technique, even in the absence of endoleak. This phenomenon is most likely due to maintenance of high pressure within the aneurysm sac, presumably by pressure transmission from the adjacent aortic lumen (1). We have postulated that, in most cases, this pressure may be transmitted through thrombus, which is acting to seal the endograft from flowing blood, but which is not an adequate barrier to totally exclude the aneurysm sac from pressure effects. However, it is likely that there are other causes of endotension, including transmission of pressure across the wall of an endograft itself, perhaps associated with high porosity or other factors.

The purpose of this chapter is to present a summary of our clinical experience in a series of cases of apparent endotension, demonstrating the presentation, investigations performed, and treatment. The chapter also presents an analysis of a range of possible causes for endotension.

I. DEFINITION OF ENDOTENSION

The following definition of endotension has previously been applied (2): "Endotension is a condition associated with endoluminal vascular grafts, defined by persistent or recurrent pressurization of an aneurysm sac after endovascular repair, without evidence of endoleak. Endotension may be presumed when there is continued growth of the aneurysm sac on progressive imaging studies, and may be proven by pressure measurements or other evidence of stress on the aneurysm wall." It should be acknowledged that many apparent cases of endotension may represent simply a missed endoleak; in such situations, an endoleak is in fact present but has not been detected on the imaging investigations performed. This may be due to a variety of factors such as early timing of computed tomography (CT) images (images late in the phase of contrast perfusion are often required to detect type II endoleak), imprecise duplex ultrasound technique, or poorly performed angiographic studies.

II. CLINICAL EXPERIENCE: CASE REPORTS

The following brief case reports demonstrate some of the difficulties in investigation and interpretation of morphological changes in the AAA sac after endovascular grafting and illustrate the evolution of concepts regarding etiology of continued pressurization of the sac contents without endoleak ("endotension") (2–4).

A. Patient 1

Mr. HF, a 71-year-old male, had successful implantation of an EVT tube graft (EndoVascular Technologies, Menlo Park, CA) for management of a 5.6 cm AAA in April 1994 (Fig. 1). Completion angiogram and predischarge CT scan both confirmed exclusion of the aneurysm sac with no evidence of endoleak. Follow-up CT scans at 6, 12, 24, and 36 months also showed no endoleak or other complications, but the maximal diameter increased from 5.6 to 7.4 cm over that period (Fig. 2). The aneurysm remained asymptomatic but was noted to be pulsatile to physical examination.

Occult endoleak was suspected, and detailed angiography was performed to search for perigraft leak (endoleak type I) or retrograde flow via lumbar or mesenteric arteries (endoleak type II). Despite directed injection and late angiographic views, no contrast could be demonstrated within the aneurysm sac. It was determined that open repair of the aneurysm was indicated; at operation the AAA sac was found to be filled with soft thrombus, which showed no evidence of absorption or contraction (Fig. 3). There was no evidence of blood flow in communication with the sac contents and no retrograde flow from any collateral vessels.

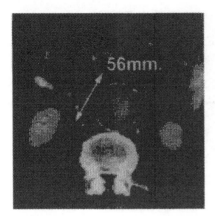

Figure 1. Preoperative CT scan of the AAA in patient 1.

Comment

This case demonstrates the extensive investigations that may be required to prove that endoleak is not present (in other cases, directed angiography has successfully shown endoleak due to patent lumbars, inferior mesenteric artery, or other causes). We suspected that pressure might be transmitted through the walls of the endograft material, through pulsatile movements of the unsupported graft wall, or through a rim of thrombus lining the exterior of

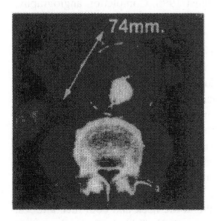

Figure 2. Progress CT scan at 24 months in patient 1 showing aneurysm enlargement without evidence of endoleak.

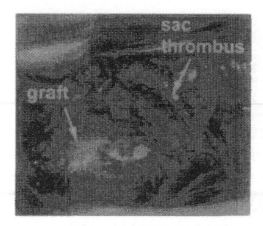

Figure 3. Patient 1: No endoleak was detected at open repair of the aneurysm. The aneurysm sac was full of soft, semi-liquid thrombus surrounding the endograft.

the graft at the proximal or distal attachment sites. Operative findings were most consistent with the latter etiology.

B. Patient 2

HF, a 68-year-old male, had successful implantation of a custom-made White-Yu bifurcated endovascular graft in August 1996. Completion angiography, discharge CT scan, and follow-up CT scans at 6 and 12 months showed exclusion of the AAA sac with no evidence of endoleak (Fig. 4). The aneurysm size initially decreased, but it had increased by 0.7 cm at the 18-month follow-up scan and had become pulsatile to physical examination. Detailed angiography showed no evidence of endoleak, but there was evidence of distal displacement of the proximal attachment wireforms by approximally 1 cm (Fig. 5). It was determined that conversion to open repair should be performed.

At operation, pressure measurements were obtained within the AAA sac by insertion of a needle attached to a pressure manometer (Fig. 6). Systolic and diastolic pressures were recorded from within the sac, external to the endovascular graft device, at the following intervals: (1) after exposure of the aneurysm, prior to application of aortic clamps, and (2) after application of proximal and distal vascular clamps to the aortic neck and both iliac arteries. Results of these pressure measurements are detailed in Table 1. The aortic sac was then opened, revealing gel-like semi-liquid thrombus within the sac, particularly

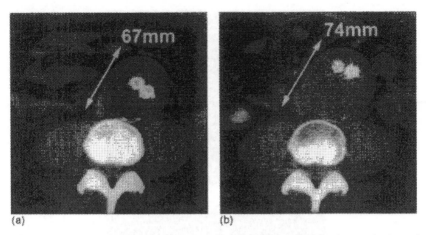

(a) (b)

Figure 4. Patient 2: (a) The CT scan 12 months after endovascular repair showed complete AAA exclusion. (b) At 24 months, CT scan documented continued AAA exclusion but aneurysm enlargement.

around the proximal attachment site (Fig. 7). This soft thrombus appeared to be the major tissue component forming a seal around the top end of the graft device.

The endovascular graft was removed and the AAA was repaired successfully with a 22 mm diameter conventional vascular graft of tube configuration. There were no significant postoperative complications.

Comment

Before application of an aortic clamp, the systolic pressure within the thrombus around the graft was identical to the systemic systolic pressure as measured from a radial arterial line. The aneurysm remained pulsatile to

Table 1. Systemic and Aneurysm Sac Pressures at Time of Conversion to Open Repair

Patient		Systemic blood pressure (mmHg)	Aneurysm sac pressure (mmHg)
2	Preclamp	140/84	138/80
	Postclamp	155/92	40/36
4	Preclamp	126/75	118/70
	Postclamp	130/79	38/33

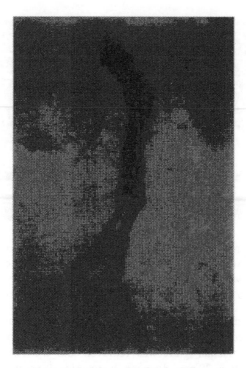

Figure 5.   Patient 2: Angiography did not reveal an endoleak; however, the proximal wireforms were displaced distally by approximately 1 cm (seen below the accessory left renal artery).

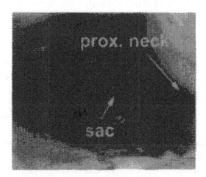

Figure 6.   Patient 2: The aneurysm sac pressure was measured by placing a needle connected to a pressure manometer into the sac.

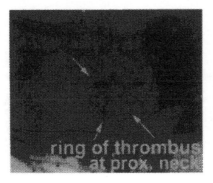

Figure 7.   Patient 2: Upon removal of the endovascular graft, a ring of thrombus was evident at the proximal neck region of the AAA.

palpation at laparotomy, and the distribution of semi-liquid thrombus around the proximal attachment site supported the fact that the proximal seal in this case was being completed by a rim of thrombus. This allowed transmission of systemic blood pressure into the aneurysm contents, with continued AAA expansion. [Measurements taken during open surgical repair of aneurysms have shown that thrombus within an aneurysm sac transmits pressure to the wall (5).]

C. Patient 3

FR, a 76-year-old male with a previous history of renal transplantation, had endovascular repair of a large 8.8 cm AAA using a custom-made bifurcated White-Yu device in August 1996. Initial follow-up imaging showed no endoleak, but follow-up imaging at 6 months showed an expansion of the AAA sac, with endoleak. CT scan and detailed angiography suggested that the leak was emanating from an iliac limb of the device, possibly from the overlap zone of the limbs with the bifurcated trunk segment (Fig. 8, top). The endograft was reinforced by implantation of two Talent iliac limbs to overlap those already present (Fig. 8, bottom). This resulted in apparent seal of the endoleak, but continued expansion of the aneurysm occurred in association with symptoms.

The patient was readmitted to hospital for treatment of severe abdominal pains at an interval of 12 months after the revision procedure. CT scan now showed contained rupture of the AAA (Fig. 9). At emergency surgery, the endograft devices were removed and large amounts of semi-liquid thrombus were noted surrounding the device components. Apart from quite minor

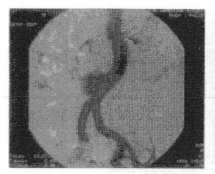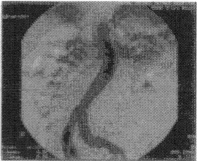

Figure 8.   Patient 3: (Left) Six months after endovascular repair there is evidence of type III endoleak from the overlap zone between graft trunk and an iliac limb. (Right) Overlap-zone endoleak was sealed by placement of two Talent iliac limbs.

retrograde bleeding from a lumbar artery, no blood was detected within the sac. Successful open repair was achieved, with continuing function of the transplant kidney.

Comment

Endoleak was confirmed in this patient in the early follow-up period. Treatment by secondary endograft procedures led to apparent closure of the endoleak, but the aneurysm continued to expand and eventually ruptured. (The relatively stable course of this patient supports a concept that bleeding from a ruptured AAA associated with endotension may be significantly reduced due to the intact graft surrounded by thrombus only.) It is also possible that rupture in this case was due to endoleak from the lumbar vessel, which was found to be patient during the operation. Emergency surgery was successful and again supported a mechanism of pressure transmission through thrombus as being significant in the etiology of this pathological process.

D. Patient 4

RL, a 73-year-old male, had successful implantation of a Vanguard bifurcated endovascular graft (Boston Scientific, Natick, MA) in November 1996. Completion angiography, discharge CT scan, and follow-up CT scans at 6, 12, 18, and 24 months showed exclusion of the AAA sac with no evidence of endoleak. The aneurysm size initially decreased but had increased by 1.6 cm at the 24-month follow-up scan and had become pulsatile to physical

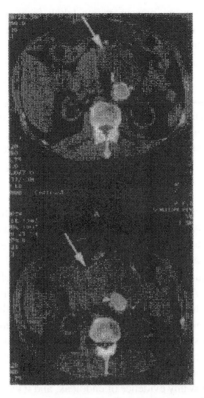

Figure 9. Patient 3: Twelve months after apparently successful secondary endoleak repair, there was evidence of contained AAA rupture (arrows).

examination. Duplex ultrasound showed no endoleak. Abdominal x-rays and angiography showed evidence of downward displacement of the proximal end of the endograft, but there was no radiological evidence of endoleak. The patient was offered secondary endograft procedure or conversion to open repair and elected to have conventional surgery.

At operation, pressure measurements were obtained from the AAA sac by similar methodology to patient 2 (see Table 1). The endograft was removed and conventional repair of the AAA by tube graft was performed.

Comment

This patient was shown to have definite slippage of the proximal attachment stents, and despite the fact that endoleak did not develop, the findings at operation and the pressure measurements taken from within the sac again supported a mechanism of pressure transmission from the aortic lumen to the AAA contents via thrombotic gel material.

E. Patient 5

PK, a 76-year-old female patient, had successful exclusion of a 5.8 cm AAA using a Vanguard bifurcated graft (Boston Scientific, Natick, MA). There were no perioperative complications, and regular imaging studies were satisfactory at all follow-up visits, showing no evidence of endoleak and progressive shrinking of the aneurysm sac. At the 3-year postoperative interval, however, the AXR showed distortion of the metallic stent framework of the device; CT scan and duplex ultrasound showed no evidence of endoleak, but there was now 6 mm enlargement of the AAA sac compared to the most recent study, 12 months prior. No further investigations or interventions were performed at this stage, but the next follow-up interval was shortened to 6 months.

At the subsequent visit (now 3.5 years postop), clinical examination revealed that the AAA had regained its pulsatility, with mild associated tenderness. Imaging studies again showed no evidence of endoleak, but there was further enlargement of the sac. Angiography was performed to determine if an endoleak had been missed, and to judge whether the situation may be salvaged by a secondary endovascular procedure to salvage the existing device (the patient remained extremely keen to avoid open operation due to risk factors). The aortogram did not show any evidence of endoleak, and it was considered that the AAA enlargement and pulsatility was most likely due to endotension.

In this case secondary endovascular graft (for relining or reinforcing the flow channel) was not considered to be a good option due to the severe distortion of the device in situ. Open operation was performed; pressures in the thrombosed AAA sac were again found to be in the systemic range. The graft was firmly secured and well sealed within the aortic neck, but both iliac limbs were only loosely applied within the orifice region of the iliac arteries, with a thrombotic lining. In addition, the modular contralateral limb was on the point of detaching from the main graft body, with the seal in this zone being essentially thrombus only. There were no fabric tears or stent fractures.

Comment

This case nicely demonstrates the relationship of device structural changes to endotension and the likely predisposition to endoleak in patients who have a thrombotic seal in a zone of device shift, dislocation, or retraction from the iliac attachment points. In several other cases in our experience, structural alterations of Vanguard grafts have resulted in detachment of one or both iliac limbs from within the iliac artery, resulting in obvious endoleak and repressurization of the sac. In the current case this process was apparently intercepted at a point before the iliac limbs had retracted sufficiently to produce endoleak, but the rim of thrombus that remained as the only sealing region was transmitting pressure into the sac. Endoleak may have been only days away. In addition, the imminent disconnection of the contralateral stump was also a site of pressure transmission. In retrospect, it would have been possible to salvage the situation by secondary implantation of new iliac limbs on both sides, with distal extensions well down into the iliac attachment zones, but there would still remain the possibility of late fabric tears in the trunk region. (It is now known that the Vanguard graft is notoriously prone to late fabric defects.) Secondary implantation of a completely new bifurcated graft may become desirable in such cases, although the device design does not lend itself to total relining with a new bifurcated graft; use of a secondary aorto-iliac graft is more feasible, but requires supplementary femoro-femoral bypass procedure.

III. DISCUSSION

Endoleak, the presence of blood flow outside the lumen of an endoluminal graft, can be detected by many forms of conventional vascular imaging, including duplex ultrasound, CT scan, MRI scan, and angiography (6). It has been demonstrated conclusively that the presence of type I attachment site endoleak will cause continued expansion of an AAA in most cases (7,8). This can lead to rupture of the aneurysm (9–12). On the other hand, type II retrograde endoleak may be associated with stable AAA size or even with shrinkage of the AAA sac in some cases (13). In other cases, persistent type II endoleak has definitely resulted in AAA enlargement. When an aneurysm is noted to increase in size [maximal diameter or volume (14)], the question must arise as to whether occult endoleak is present. This has certainly been so in a number of other cases in our experience—AAA enlargement was observed on CT scans that did not show endoleak, but endoleak was later shown to be present by means of ultrasound or angiography. In the cases presented above, however, extensive investigations were performed in a search for occult endoleak that had not been demonstrated on routine follow-up studies. Endoleak may be missed on CT scan if the images are obtained early in the cycle after infusion of the vascular contrast medium; late CT images should also be obtained to demonstrate retrograde flow from collateral arteries or delayed blood flow in the AAA sac occurring through the graft wall (type III) or through small channels around the ends of the graft (type I).

The cases reported above illustrate the fact that aneurysms can continue to expand without endoleak and support the theory that this is often due to high pressures within the aneurysm sac being transmitted through a layer of thrombus or semi-liquid thrombotic gel. In the three cases where intrasac pressures were measured, the systolic pressures within the thrombus were similar to systemic pressures. This finding, along with the experience of others, led to the concept of "endotension." The presence of the endograft and the thrombotic seal at attachment site in the majority of these reported cases were doing nothing to reduce pressures leading to continued expansion of the AAA.

A. Pressure Measurements

Several groups have measured pressures within the aneurysm through a catheter adjacent to the endovascular graft (15–17). Chuter et al. (16) demonstrated that exclusion of an aneurysm by endovascular graft leads to a significant reduction of intrasac pressures; mean aneurysm pressure was 36.5/33.8 mmHg compared to mean radial arterial pressures of 118.5/50.5 mmHg. These findings corresponded with a reduction in the palpable pulse and an absence of perigraft flow on follow-up CT scans. On the other hand, Stelter and coworkers (17) showed, using similar methodology, that intra-aneurysmal pressures remained high when endoleak channels occurred. Noninvasive methods of measuring intra-aneurysmal pressures are not yet available; Malina et al. (18) have suggested that an indirect indication may be obtained from ultrasound monitoring of aortic wall pulsatility. Implantable transducers are being developed and may provide useful information regarding the changing pressure environment within the AAA sac, the effects of various factors on sac pressures, and the relationship between AAA pressure and growth.

B. Mechanisms of AAA Growth

The mechanisms leading to continued aneurysm growth despite evidence of radiographic exclusion have not been elucidated. It is logical to assume that a contributing factor is transmission of systemic blood pressure. However, an increase in sac volume cannot occur without accumulation of more luminal content. Ongoing thrombus accumulation suggests circulatory inflow, but no outflow. "Endotension" may represent a form of endoleak so slow that blood clots at the source of leakage. Ongoing degradative processes in the arterial wall may be an additional mechanism of sac growth by wall thinning. It is conceivable that this may be related to enzymatic activity in retained thrombus, which is removed during open aneurysm repair. However, degradative processes alone cannot cause sac enlargement; there must also be pressure and accumulation of new luminal material to expand the increase in volume.

Pressure transmission may be through the wall of the graft (porous graft fabrics or defects in the fabric material), through thrombus "sealing" an endoleak, or through thrombus lining the attachment site. Graft material has previously been implicated in build-up of serious fluid by transudation through a PTFE graft used at open repair of AAA (19). Deployment of an endograft low in the aortic neck or later displacement of the proximal attachment segment may be causative factors for endotension due to pressure transmission through a lining or rim of thrombus and may represent an intermediate stage in the development of attachment site endoleak—this pathogenesis seemed likely in four of the cases reported herein.

C. Relevance of Endotension to Clinical Practice

There are several significant implications to be drawn from this experience:

1. Noninvasive pressure-monitoring systems are required. At present, pressures within an AAA or within the sac of an AAA after endografting can only be obtained by invasive means, using a direct pressure line.
2. Radiographic seal of endoleak may be achieved by thrombus, which may not reduce the pressures within the AAA. Imaging studies may therefore convey a false sense of security regarding the effectiveness of treatments for endoleak.
3. Continued long-term monitoring of AAA size and/or volume is essential, in addition to studies that demonstrate the presence or absence of endoleak.
4. Experience to date would suggest that the presence of high pressure within the AAA sac without endoleak is relatively uncommon. In our series, this has been detected in only 7 of more than 400 patients treated by endovascular grafts. Nevertheless, late changes in graft structure or position may predispose to an increasing incidence with time.

One aspect that still requires investigation is whether pressure reduction within the aneurysm sac is achieved as effectively when the seal of small channels in the graft wall is thrombotic rather than structural; thrombus (or fibrin plug) sealing a flow channel may transmit higher pressures to the interior of the aneurysm sac leading to different pressure effects on the aortic wall in both the early and late stages. Intriguing data have been produced by Marty et al. (20), who demonstrated that in in vitro studies, embolization of endoleak channels by coils, while achieving angiographic seal, did not lower intra-aneurysmal pressure. There may be differences in pressure transmission through holes or pores of various sizes because of variances in sealing efficacy by thrombus (21). These variances may lead to a differential tendency for an aneurysm sac to shrink or perhaps to enlarge.

D. Causes of Endotension

Endotension appears to be the result of maintained high pressure in the excluded AAA sac due to transmission through the wall of the endograft, around its ends at the attachment zones, or by accumulation of fluid within the sac. It is also possible that an aneurysm may enlarge under the influence of factors other than pressure (22).

Since noninvasive monitoring of pressures within the aneurysm sac is not yet available; endotension must often be inferred from growth of the sac over time intervals of 6 months or so; if the aneurysm remains pulsatile to physical examination, it is supportive clinical evidence for the presence of high pressure within the sac. It remains unknown whether high pressure is the only mechanism of continued AAA growth after endovascular grafting. It is possible that sac enlargement may occur under the influence of other factors, such as the accumulation of material within the AAA sac, transudation or exudation through the fabric of the prosthetic graft, transmission of pressure throughout the aneurysm sac influenced by graft wall movements or oscillations (18), genetically modulated activity within the sac thrombus, or other unknown factors.

In a recent paper Risberg et al. (23) presented a report of 4 patients who developed endotension after AAA repair procedures (1 after open repair and 3 cases after endovascular AAA repair), and they described the finding of clear fluid within the aneurysm sac (found at open exploration in one patient, and by percutaneous aspiration in 3 patients). They proposed an alternative mechanism for causation of endotension in some cases involving in situ build-up of excess fluid around the graft and eventual formation of a "hygroma." A possible primary mechanism of hyperfibrinolysis within the thrombus of the sac was proposed. In contrast to previous reports, the pressures within the sac in their patients were nonpulsatile and significantly lower (approximately half) than the systemic blood pressure.

This proposed mechanism for continued sac expansion due to fluid accumulation within the sac had previously been postulated (2,4,19). The report of Risberg et al. (23) provided valuable supportive evidence for those previous concepts and also gave guidance on the possibility of diagnosis of intra-sac hygroma by CT scan (the attenuation on CT was significantly less in the AAA sac than in the graft lumen, as measured by Hounsfield units).

It is interesting to speculate on the possible role of graft material in the etiology of this build-up of fluid around the graft (3 of the 4 cases were related to PTFE grafts, which are notoriously prone to external build-up of seroma fluid in some patients undergoing hemodialysis). Fluid transudate across PTFE graft wall may be an important factor. A similar previous case after open AAA repair using a PTFE graft was reported in 1998 (19). Furthermore, it would appear that in the absence of endoleak, the only way for fluid to accumulate within the sac would be by transmission of fluid across the graft wall or across the wall of the AAA. We have proposed previously that an intermittent or very low-flow endoleak would also provoke fluid build-up (2).

E. Possible Alternative Mechanisms of Endotension

There are a number of possible mechanisms for endotension (Table 2) (22). Pressure may remain high in the excluded AAA sac due to transmission through a rim of thrombus at or around the ends or attachment zones of the prosthesis; in previous experience this has been particularly associated with slip or displacement of the proximal aspect of the graft (2). This situation would appear to be a precursor to development of late type I endoleak. In some cases a small endoleak channel may recurrently develop and rethrombose, each time with accumulation of additional material within the sac. Undetected endoleak may also be present but not detected on present imaging techniques, particularly if the flow is very low.

Fluid and pressure transmission through the wall or fabric of the endograft may occur with graft materials that are highly porous, or through holes in the graft at the site of sutures or wireforms that penetrate the fabric. In some cases, persistence of such small tears has been shown to cause late "microleaks" through the graft wall (24). Graft materials, weave patterns, or porosity may also be important in determining transudation, ultrafiltration, or exudation of fluid components of serum from within the graft lumen into the AAA sac.

If pressure build-up is entirely due to a mechanism of in situ production and accumulation of fluid within the sac, one must consider how this may occur without fluid shift from other spaces. Enzymatic or fibrinolytic activity may certainly contribute to this process by lysis of thrombus within the sac, but it would still seem to require some active transport or secretion of material from without. An infective process may lead to such local activity.

Table 2. Possible Mechanisms of Endotension

1. *Pressure Transmission to AAA Sac Around Ends of Graft*
    Layer of thrombus between graft and aortic wall (or iliac artery wall)
    Graft displacement exposing layer of thrombus at aortic neck
    Endoleak channel sealed by thrombus
    Undetected endoleak
    Intermittent endoleak channel
    Very low-flow endoleak channel

2. *Pressure Transmission Through Wall of Graft*
    High graft porosity
    Microleak through graft interstices
    Transudate of fluid through graft fabric
    Exudate of fluid through graft fabric
    Graft pulsatility/wall movements

3. *Pressure Transmission from Branch Vessels*
    Thrombus over orifice of IMA or lumbars

4. *Pressure Build-Up from Fluid Accumulation In Situ*
    Graft infection
    Thrombus fibrinolysis/hygroma
    Genetic modulation
    Enzymatic activity
    Others

5. *AAA Enlargement Without Raised Pressure*
    Genetic modulation
    Enzymatic activity
    ?Graft infection
    ?Growth factors
    Others

Finally, growth of an AAA sac may be independent of pressure, perhaps under the influence of genetic modulation or growth factors leading to hyperplasia or hypertrophy of elements of the aortic wall.

IV. CONCLUSIONS

Ideally, successful endovascular repair of aneurysms would reliably result in shrinkage and contraction of the aneurysm sac. In practice, however, some aneurysms remain static in size, whereas others enlarge. Increase in size of the aneurysm potentially exposes the treated patient to an ongoing risk of aneurysm rupture, even if the pressure within is not particularly high. Endotension is now recognized as an association with slipped or misplaced endografts in situations where flow into the sac is being prevented only by a barrier of thrombus, which potentially transmits systemic pressure to the sac and which may be a precursor to type I endoleak or other complications. Other causes are possible and may be related to factors in device design and construction. Treatment options include secondary endograft implantation, including cuffs or extension limbs, as well as conversion to open repair. Implanted pressure transducers may help provide further information on the occurrence and outcome of endotension cases in the near future. It is likely that many years of basic research and clinical observation will be required to fully elucidate the nature and behavior or this unusual phenomenon.

REFERENCES

1. White GH, May J, Waugh RC, Chaufour X, Yu W. Type III and Type IV Endoleak: Towards a complete definition of blood flow in the sac after endoluminal AAA repair. J Endovasc Surg 1998; 5:305–309.
2. White GH, May J, Waugh RC, Stephen MS, Harris JP. Endotension: An explanation for continued AAA growth after successful endoluminal repair. J Endovasc Surg 1999; 6:308–315.
3. Gilling-Smith G, Brennan J, Harris PL, Bakran A, Gould D, McWilliams R. Endotension: Definition, classification and implications for surveillance and intervention after endovascular aneurysm repair. J Endovasc Surgery 1999; 6:305–307.
4. White GH, May J. How should endotension be defined? History of a concept and evolution of a term. J Endovasc Surg 2000; 7:435–438.
5. Schurink GWH, van Baalen JM, Visser MJT, van Bockel JH. Thrombus within an aortic aneurysm does not reduce pressure on the aneurysm wall. J Vasc Surg 2000; 31:501–506.
6. White GH, Yu W, May J, Chaufour X, Stephen MS. Endoleak as a complication of endoluminal grafting of abdominal aortic aneurysms: Classification, incidence, diagnosis and management. J Endovasc Surg 1997; 4:152–168.
7. May J, White GH, Yu W, Waugh RC, Stephen MS, Harris JP. A prospective study of changes in morphology and dimensions of abdominal aortic aneurysms following endoluminal repair: A preliminary report. J Endovasc Surg 1995; 2:343–347.

8. Matsumura JS, Pearce WH, McCarthy WJ, Yao JS. Reduction in aortic aneurysm size: early results after endovascular graft placement. J Vasc Surg 1997; 25:113–123.

9. Parodi JC. Endovascular repair of abdominal aortic aneurysms and other arterial lesions. J Vasc Surg 1995; 21:549–557.

10. Lumsden AB, Allen RC, Chaikof EL, et al. Delayed rupture of aortic aneurysms following endovascular stent grafting. Am J Surg 1995; 170:174–178.

11. White GH, Yu W, May J, Waugh RC, Chaufour X, Harris JP, Stephen MS. Three-year experience with the White-Yu endovascular GAD graft for transluminal repair of aortic and iliac aneurysms. J Endovasc Surg 1997; 4:124–136.

12. Torsello GB, Klenk E, Kasprzak B, Umsheid T. Rupture of abdominal aortic aneurysm previously treated by endovascular stentgraft. J Vasc Surg 1998; 28:184–187.

13. Resch T, Ivancev K, Lindh M, Nyman U, Brunkwall J, Malina M, Lindblad B. Persistent collateral perfusion of abdominal aortic aneurysm after endovascular repair does not lead to progressive change in aneurysm diameter. J Vasc Surg 1998; 28:242–249.

14. Singh-Ranger R, McArthur T, Raphael M, Lees W, Adiseshiah M. What happens to abdominal; aortic aneurysms after endovascular grafting? A volumetric study using spiral CT angiography. J Intervent Radiol 1998; 13:145–146.

15. Sanchez LA, Faries PL, Marin ML, Ohki T, Parsons RE, Marty B, Soeiro D, Olivieri S, Veith FJ, et al. Chronic intraaneurysmal pressure measurement: an experimental method for evaluating the effectiveness of endovascular aneurysm exclusion. J Vasc Surg 1997; 26:222–230.

16. Chuter T, Ivancev K, Malina M, Resch T, Brunkwall J, Lindblad B, Risberg B. Aneurysm pressure following aneurysm exclusion. Eur J Vasc Endovasc Surg 1997; 13:85–87.

17. Stelter W, Umscheid T, Ziegler P. Three-year experience with modular stent-graft devices for endovascular AAA treatment. J Endovasc Surg 1997; 4:362–369.

18. Malina M, Lanne T, Ivancev K, Lindblad B, Brunkwall J. Reduced pulsatile wall motion of abdominal aortic aneurysms after endovascular repair. J Vasc Surg 1998; 27:624–631.

19. Williams GM. The management of massive ultrafiltration distending the aneurysm sac after abdominal aortic aneurysm repair with a polytetrafluoro-ethylene aortobiiliac graft. J Vasc Surg 1998; 28:551–555.

20. Marty B, Sanchez LA, Ohki T, Wain RA, Faries PL, Cynamon J, Marin ML, Veith FJ. Endoleak after endovascular graft repair of experimental aortic aneurysms: does coil embolization with angiographic "seal" lower intraaneurysmal pressure? J Vasc Surg 1998; 27:454–462.

21. Mehta M, Ohki T, Veith FJ, Lipsitz EC. All sealed endoleaks are not the same: a treatment strategy based on an ex vivo analysis. Eur J Endovasc Surg 2001; 21:541–544.

22. White GH. What are the causes of endotension? J Endovasc Ther 2001; 8:454–456.

23. Risberg B, Delle M, Eriksson E, Klingenstierna H, Lonn L. Aneurysmal sac hygroma: a cause of endotension. J Endovasc Ther 2001; 8:447–453.

24. Matsumura JS, Ryu RK, Ouriel K. Identification and implications of transgraft microleaks after endovascular repair of aortic aneurysms. J Vasc Surg 2001; 34:190–197.

7

Experience, Views, and Management of Endoleaks with the Zenith Endoluminal Graft for Abdominal Aortic Aneurysm

Michael M. D. Lawrence-Brown
Royal Perth Hospital, Perth, Western Australia, Australia

James B. Semmens
University of Western Australia, Nedlands, Western Australia, Australia

John L. Anderson
Ashford Hospital, Adelaide, South Australia, Australia

I. INTRODUCTION

Advances in medical and imaging technology in the 1990s has seen the introduction and rapid increase in the use of endoluminal stent grafting as an attractive and elegant alternative treatment modality for the treatment of aneurysm of the abdominal aorta (AAA) (1–6). This technology is much less invasive with reduced stress upon the patient, which is reflected in the 30-day mortality of 1.8% for 277 bifurcated endografts (7). The risk-benefit analysis of this procedure is determined more by the morphology of the aneurysm rather than by the fitness of the patient for surgery, success being determined by the ability of the device to immediately and permanently exclude the aneurysm chamber from the expansive forces of blood flow (6). Most endografts can be inserted with minimal stress under general anaesthetic, epidural, or even local anaesthetic: blood loss is minimal, ICU admission unnecessary, and postoperative care similar to hernia repair. Only successfully excluded aneurysms will diminish in size and cease to pose a risk of rupture (7). While the evolution of endoluminal technology warrants confidence in its future as an alternate treatment modality for aneurysm repair, fundamental questions remain about the long-term safety and efficacy of these devices (4). The term endoleak was coined by Geoff White to describe the observation of flow within the sac of an aneurysm through which an endoluminal graft had been placed (8). Its important implication is that the aneurysm sac is still pressurized to a greater or lesser extent. It is a subset of pressurized aneurysm sacs following endoluminal grafting. If flow is detected, pressure is implied, and until recently this was the only method of verifying continued pressurized aneurysms. An endoleak, being a mark of failure of objective, is the Achilles' heel of endoluminal grafting.

The Zenith Endoluminal Stent Graft Program (Zenith ELG Program) was initiated at Royal Perth Hospital (Western Australia) in 1993 for the treatment of AAA disease, and the Zenith Endograft is currently used in 87% of the endoluminal cases for AAA in Australasia (Australia and New Zealand), as well as across northern Europe and Asia (Fig. 1). The aim of the Zenith ELG Program is to provide information that will contribute to the development of guidelines for best practice in the use of endoluminal stent grafts, provide an infrastructure tool for the assessment of clinical outcomes and device performance, provide a basis for quality assurance and audit activities, and regulatory policy. The Zenith Research Program encompasses the collaboration of the Centre for Health Services Research (University of Western Australia) to provide data collection and outcomes data and the CSIRO to further evaluate the forces acting on an endoluminal graft and blood flow parameters. The multidisciplinary team provides an ideal environment for further research to address the concerns and will be applicable to understanding the performance of all types of grafts.

The Zenith ELG Research Database was established in 1998 to include comprehensive data for 322 patients who were treated with endoluminal repair for AAA from 18 endoluminal centers in Australasia between August 4, 1994, and December 31, 1998. The data collected on each patient included demographic information, device characteristics, risk factors, comorbidities, anatomical information, radiological data [from sources including plain abdominal x-rays, computerized axial computed tomography (CT) scans and angiograms taken before, during, and following surgery], and clinical and radiological follow-up information. The follow-up protocol included clinical examination, biochemical testing, abdominal CT scan, and plain abdominal x-ray within 30 days, at 6 months, and then annually thereafter. If the CT scan was not performed prior to discharge for clinical or logistic reasons, a duplex Doppler

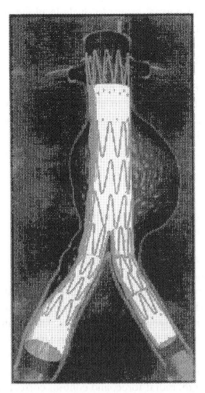

Figure 1. The Zenith bifurcated endoluminal graft for aneurysm of the abdominal aorta is shown in the accompanying diagram and used by the authors. The experience and data formulate the views presented.

ultrasound was performed pending the CT scan. Information was located at a central office in the Centre for Health Service Research, The University of Western Australia. All CT scans were reviewed by a single observer for this study. This database has provided us with a basis for determining and analyzing the cause and effects of endoleaks, most of which are non–device-specific.

II. ENDOLEAK

The security and durability of an endoluminal graft is dependent upon the forces that anchor it in place and the mechanisms that maintain wall contact between the graft and normal artery to exclude blood flow from around or through the stent graft, into the aneurysm chamber (7,9,10). Endoleaks were divided into four categories by White et al. (8), with the recent addition of endoleak caused by endotension:

1. Type I is the direct flow of blood from the aorta into the chamber of the aneurysm and is due to an inadequate proximal (Type Ia) and distal (Type Ib) seal between the graft and the wall of the artery.
2. Type II endoleak is when blood, which has originated from branch vessels (inferior mesenteric artery or lumbar artery) with retrograde flow, flows into the chamber of the aneurysm.
3. Type III is due to failure of the graft with disruption of the materials or structure.
4. Type IV is due to fabric porosity.
5. Type V is due to endotension.

Types I and III are the most dangerous because they enable the full force of the blood flow to be exerted upon the arterial wall.

Proximal endoleak is the most dangerous because the options for treatment are fewer (Figs. 2 and 3). The causes are inadequate wall contact for 360° due to contour changes affecting wall contact, and waists or mural projections, which hold the stent away from the arterial wall. Short necks fail to provide sufficient wall contact for seal, and angulation affects both of the above. Some corrections have been possible with additional stents to increase wall contact with length, radial force, and contour correction to force back the projection and with better wall contact with the use of proximal extension when deployment has been lower than intended (9). Late proximal endoleaks have been due to poor patient selection and stent migration. Examples of poor patient selection have been due to large-diameter necks, which have continued to expand with significant rimmed thrombus lining the neck and precluding adequate wall attachment.

Stent migration is a cause of endoleak, especially late endoleaks, as the sac becomes exposed to aortic pressure once more. The Gianturco stent was modified after February 1996 to provide a more secure and durable attachment system. Traction testing demonstrates that the dislodgment force is increased approximately 10-fold from friction alone by the use of attachment hooks (7).

Distal endoleaks have been due to length-assessment problems with deployment short of the intended landing zone, thus not achieving adequate seal, and in two cases of fabric damage. One case of fabric damage was due to balloon disruption and the second due to throwing back of the fabric with

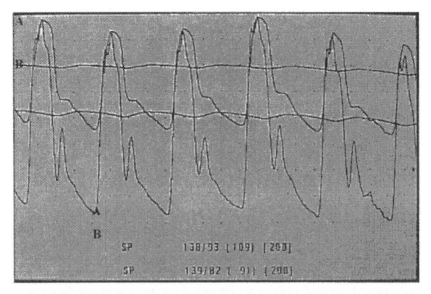

Figure 2. Pressure changes showing higher mean pressure and prolonged pulse wave in the false lumen of a dissected aorta with inflow and restricted outflow, similar to a type I proximal endoleak.

manipulation. Distal endoleaks may be sealed more readily by extension pieces, including extension down into the external iliac arteries.

The third category is termed retroleak. These occur because of persistent collaterals into the aneurysm chamber, namely, the inferior mesenteric artery (IMA) and lumbar vessels. The IMA has been persistently patent in five cases. Two sealed within one year and intervention was not necessary. In two patients the IMA was occluded using microcatheters and in one by the application of a liga-clip because of evidence of enlarging rather than contracting aneurysms. No lumbar vessels have needed occlusion in this series. Persistent endoleaks due to retroleaks is an area that still needs clarification.

III. OBJECTIVE ASSESSMENT OF DESIRED OUTCOMES

The indication to seal a persistent inferior mesenteric artery retroleak, particularly if they are large vessels, is expansion rather than contraction of the

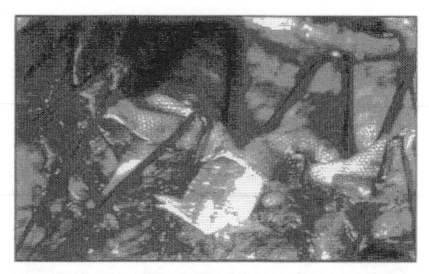

Figure 3. Postoperative rupture showing proximal endoleak due to an inadequate wall contact because of a relatively short neck, forshortened further on the posterior wall due to angulation, such that the covered stent can be seen falling into the aneurysm sac, with the marker arrow placed through the channel from neck to aneurysm sac.

aneurysm. For static aneurysms, the decision is based on continued observation. The method of occlusion may be endovascular, as described above, or via a minor procedure to apply a clip to the origin of the vessel. In the medium and longer term, shrinkage of the aneurysm sac is the best indicator of successful treatment.

CT is the current internationally accepted modality in the follow-up of endoluminal grafting for AAA and currently used as the standard procedure. However, the Perth-based experience is that color duplex ultrasound provides a much less invasive and much more cost-effective means of evaluation endoluminal grafts for abdominal aortic aneurysm compared with CT scanning. While duplex ultrasound was accurate for detection of endoleaks, duplex ultrasound was more sensitive and was particularly valuable in the detection of retroleaks (Fig. 4). It is highly likely that the future direction of the ELSG program will preferentially use the less arduous duplex ultrasound procedure rather than CT for follow-up. A brief description of the advantages of Doppler ultrasound is provided below.

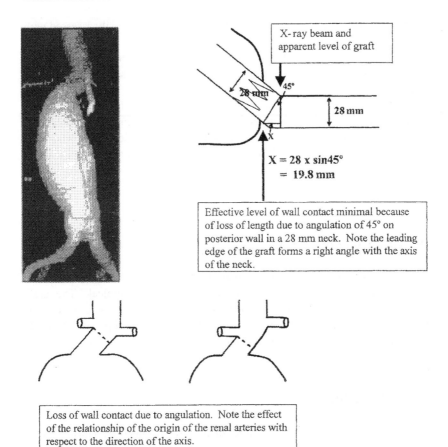

X-ray beam and apparent level of graft

45°

28 mm

28 mm

$$X = 28 \times \sin 45°$$
$$= 19.8 \text{ mm}$$

Effective level of wall contact minimal because of loss of length due to angulation of 45° on posterior wall in a 28 mm neck. Note the leading edge of the graft forms a right angle with the axis of the neck.

Loss of wall contact due to angulation. Note the effect of the relationship of the origin of the renal arteries with respect to the direction of the axis.

Figure 4. The effect of neck angulation, causing foreshortening on the posterior wall as in the case provided in Figure 3. (CT image courtesy of M. Goodman.)

Two-dimensional B-mode imaging will show the position of the graft and any twisting or kinking that may cause mechanical obstruction to the flow better than CT, and for twisting of a graft, ultrasound is better than plain x-ray or CT scan for visualizing this problem.

Color and pulsed Doppler is used to detect leaks into the aneurysm sac from the graft seals and joins. It is also better for detecting retrograde flow into the aneurysm from small arteries. Typically, flow from these sources is slow and is not seen on CT scan unless time-delay techniques are used. Normal outflow from the graft into the iliac and femoral arteries is easily assessed with pulsed Doppler.

Difficulties arise in obese patients or in patients where overlying bowel prevents good ultrasound access to the graft. In these cases spiral CT scans with intravenous contrast are appropriate.

Duplex ultrasound will not miss a major endoleak. It should be part of follow-up and considered in preference to CT, which can then be used as a back-up investigation. Routine follow-up for a 60-year-old patient who lives for 20 years having annual CT scans involves a large cost and a significant x-ray dose. Duplex ultrasound with plain x-ray should be considered for the routine check once the evaluation period is declared over.

IV. GRAFT POROSITY

With the Zenith graft, any contrast seen flowing into the aneurysm sac at the postprocedural angiogram is deemed evidence of an endoleak. The graft material is woven dacron twill-weave, and while there is some porosity and bleeding may be affected by heparization, this effect should persist no longer than would be expected for open surgery using this graft material.

V. ENDOTENSION

The term endotension has been used since it was defined by Gilling-Smith in 1999 (11). It recognizes that an aneurysm may be pressurized in the absence of being able to demonstrate flow within the sac (Fig. 5). This may appear common sense or simple physics, since flow and pressure, while they may be related, are different parameters. The obvious example that has been appreciated for many years is the demonstration of a flow current through laminated thrombus leading to an apparent normal angiogram despite the presence of an aneurysm. Placing a covered stent over a short segment of this flow current, within the sac, would fail to convince anyone that the aneurysm had been adequately treated and/or excluded. Placing an endograft that fails to completely transverse the aneurysm is the same as the above.

Endotension, or the sac pressure, is the crux of what leads to rupture, and its elimination the objective. The problems relate to its detection, monitoring, and measurement. The diagnosis of endotension continues to be a challenge: it

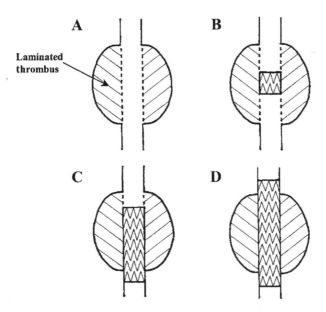

Figure 5. Only scenario D provides adequate aneurysm protection from pressure, while all may provide a similar image for the flow patterns on contrast angiography (or CT).

may not be due to blood pressure—dangerous in itself—it may be due to infection of abscess formation.

VI. UNDERSTANDING THE PHYSICS

Despite the national and international success of endoluminal repair, endovascular technology is still under development, and many important questions need to be addressed (7). The endoluminal graft must hang like a chandelier, or stand like a pillar, into the chamber of the aneurysm for a number of years, until the aneurysm shrinks to encase the graft within the chamber and provide the full-length body support enjoyed by the open repair. Constant pounding and erosion forces work to disrupt and dislodge the graft within the chamber. The long-term results of endoluminal repair are dependent on suitable morphology of the aneurysm of the abdominal aorta and an understanding of the forces that might cause an endograft to fail (12). This information will both enhance the development of the design of the endoluminal stent graft and contribute to clinical guidelines for patient selection. A balance between necessary structural strength and miniaturization is required, and the pivotal point should be determined.

REFERENCES

1. Parodi JC, Palmaz JC, Barone HD. Transfemoral infraluminal graft implantation for abdominal aortic aneurysms. Ann Vasc Surg 1991; 5:491–499.
2. Lawrence-Brown MMD, Hartley D, MacSweeny S, Kelsey P, Ives F, Holden A, Gordon M, Goodman MA, Sieunarine K. The Perth Endoluminal Bifurcated Graft System—development and early experience. J Cardiovasc Surg 1996; 4:706–712.
3. Gordon M, Lawrence-Brown MMD, Hartley D, Sieunarine K, Holden A, MacSweeney S, Hellings M. A self-expanding endoluminal graft for treatment of aneurysms: results through the development phase. Aust NZ Surg 1996; 66:621–625.
4. Harris PL, Buth J, Mialhe C, Myhre HO, Norgren L. The need for clinical trials of endovascular abdominal aortic aneurysm stent-graft repair: The EUROSTAR Project. J Endovasc Surg 1997; 4:72–77.
5. Lawrence-Brown M, Sieunarine K, Hartley D, Van Schie G, Goodman M, Prendergast F. The Perth HL-B Bifurcated Endoluminal Graft: a review of the experience and intermediate results. J Cardiovasc Surg 1998; 6:220–225.
6. Stanley B, Semmens JB, Mai Q, Goodman M, Wilkinson C, Hartley David, Lawrence-Brown MMD. Evaluation of patient selection guidelines for endoluminal grafting of aneurysm of the abdominal aorta with the Zenith graft: the Australasian experience. J Endovasc Ther 2001; 8:457–464.
7. Lawrence-Brown, MMD, Semmens, JB, Hartley, DE, Mun, RP, van Schie, G, Goodman, MA, Prendergast, FJ, Sieunarine, K. How is durability related to patient selection and graft design with endoluminal grafting for abdominal aortic aneurysm? In: Greenhalgh, RM, ed. Durability of Vascular and Endovascular Surgery. Philadelphia: W.B. Saunders, 1999:375–385.
8. White GH, Yu W, May J, et al. Endoleak as a complication of endoluminal grafting of abdominal aortic aneurysms: classification, incidence, diagnosis, and management. J Endovasc Surg 1997; 4:152–168.
9. Lawrence-Brown, MMD, Semmens, JB, Stanley, BM, Liffman, K, Bui, A, Rudman, M, Hartley, DE, et al. Endoluminal building of the aortic grafts for abdominal aortic aneurysm disease. In: Greenhalgh, RM, ed. Vascular and Endovascular Opportunities. Philadelphia: W.B. Saunders, 2000:249–261.
10. Lawrence-Brown, MMD, Semmens, JB, Hartley, DE, et al. The Zenith endoluminal stent-graft system: suprarenal fixation, safety features, modular components, fenestration and custom crafting. In: Greenhalgh, RM, ed. Vascular

and Endovascular Surgical Techniques. 4th ed. Philadelphia: W.B. Saunders, 2001:219–223.

11. Gilling-Smith G, Brennan J, Harris P, Bakran A, Gould D, McWilliams R. Endotension after endovascular aneurysm repair: definition, classification, and strategies for surveillance and intervention. J Endovasc Surg 1999; 6:305–307.

12. Liffman K, Lawrence-Brown MMD, Semmens JB, Bui A, Rudman M, Hartley D. Analytical modelling and numerical simulation of forces in an endoluminal graft. J Endovasc Ther 2001; 8:358–371.

8

Endoleak and Endotension: The Buenos Aires Perspective

Juan Carlos Parodi
University of Buenos Aires and Cardiovascular Institute of Buenos Aires, Buenos Aires, Argentina

Luis Mariano Ferreira
Cardiovascular Institute of Buenos Aires, Buenos Aires, Argentina

I. DEFINITION

Endovascular repair of abdominal aortic aneurysms (AAAs) is rapidly becoming an accepted alternative to conventional open surgical procedures, especially for high-risk patients (1–3). Despite the decreased invasiveness of the endovascular technique, numerous unique complications occurred with this new approach that were never considered an issue in conventional surgery. First and foremost among these complications was endoleak, defined as the presence of intra-aneurysm flow around an endovascular graft (4). This flow produces an increase in the pressure inside the aneurysmal sac that potentially maintains aneurysm expansion and eventually results in rupture. Although the causes of endoleak are many, any exposure of the residual aneurysm sac to arterial flow represents a potential persistent pressurization of the aneurysm and the consequent potential risk of rupture. However, the natural history of endoleaks remains poorly defined. If no endoleak is present, then the aneurysm should be maximally protected and risk of expansion or rupture minimized. Despite this concern, in some patients with endoleaks the aneurysm continues to shrink even with residual blood flow, conversely, although very rarely, aneurysms are seen to grow even in the absence of any detectable endoleak; in this latter situation the condition is named endotension or pressure endoleak. Nevertheless, the exact hemodynamic forces applied to the aneurysm sac, independent of the presence or absence of endoleak, remain poorly defined.

II. DIAGNOSIS

Endoleak can be detected by many forms of conventional vascular imaging, including duplex ultrasound, computed tomography (CT) scan, magnetic resonance imaging (MRI), and angiography. Endoleak may be missed on CT scans if the images are obtained early in the cycle after infusion of the vascular contrast medium. Late CT images should be obtained to demonstrate retrograde flow from collateral arteries or delayed blood flow into the sac through the graft wall (type IV) or anchoring sites (type I). The effects of an endoleak depend on indirect evaluation of intrasac pressure, that is, observation of changes in aneurysm diameter and/or volume.

Endoleaks may result from an incomplete seal at the graft ends or between segments, thrombus interposition between the endograft and the wall of the neck(s), incomplete deployment, or inappropriate sizing of the endograft. There may be flow through the graft material itself via interstices, tears, or perforations. Peri-graft flow may develop over time due to changes in the geometry of the endograft or/and the recipient artery due to neck dilatation, migration of the device, or aneurysmal remodeling after shrinkage. Finally non–graft-related endoleaks may be seen with retrograde flow from patent lumber or inferior mesenteric arteries.

The presence of endoleaks without enlargement and enlargement without demonstrable endoleaks (endotension) allowed us to justify our concept of aneurysm sac pressurization as a real cause of enlargement, ultimately leading to aneurysm rupture. In 1993 we treated a patient who in 1992 was the recipient of an endograft to exclude his AAA. The patient had a type I endoleak that sealed spontaneously. After 7 months the patient presented with a ruptured aneurysm. What we found in surgery prompted us to consider the concept of pressure transmission through the thrombus; no active bleeding was found inside the sac, but the gap between the endograft and the neck of the aneurysm was filled with thrombus.

Aneurysm expansion has been reported after technically successful exclusion associated with inadequate reduction of intra-aneurysmal pressure (7,8). On the other hand, not all endoleaks produce aneurysm enlargement (9,10). Some authors have reported delayed rupture in patients "waiting" for endoleak repair (11–13), while sac shrinkage with type I, II, or III endoleaks has also been described (14).

Probably consequences of endoleaks can better explained by introducing other variables to the equation of pressure and volumes:

1. Material inside the sac is often nonhomogeneous areas of fluid, sometimes with solid organized thrombus and sometimes with soft friable atheromatous material or thrombus; this can mean that pressure distribution inside the sac can be nonhomogeneous.

2. Wall thickness and resistance to dilatation varies from one patient to other. Atrophy of the wall that can result from an effective exclusion may represent a drawback for the patient in the case of occurrence of a late endoleak.

3. The larger aneurysm, the more tension of the wall. A small increase of pressure in a large aneurysm can induce a significant increase in wall tension, and, conversely, a high pressure inside a small aneurysm can be much better tolerated.

4. Amount of peri-graft flow will depend on the resulting pressurization of the sac. It is crucial, as we have proven in our experimental study, to know the amount of inflow and outflow to define the impact of the endoleak on the aneurysmal sac.

5. Size of the peri-graft channel(s): pressure per unit of surface can explain that channels with the same pressure inside can have quite different effects on the sac. It is obvious that a narrow channel will produce less effect in a nonhomogeneous sac than a large channel.

6. Systemic blood pressure is known to have an influence on the outcome of patients treated by endoluminal approach.

In an experimental model (Fig. 1) we demonstrated that in the control group (absence of endoleak) the systemic systolic pressure remained higher than the intrasac systolic pressure. The intrasac diastolic pressure in the control group was lower than the systemic diastolic pressure ($p = 0.001$). (Fig. 2) The intrasac pressure curve was damped compared with the systemic pressure curve. We also found that the presence of an endoleak causes a significant increase in aneurysm pressure (mean and diastolic pressure), the extent of which is directly proportional to the endoleak size (Fig. 3). Perhaps the most important finding of our study was that even a small size endoleak causes considerable pressure in the aneurysm sac, which in the clinical setting could lead to aneurysm rupture. As an explanation we can speculate that the blind end of the aneurysm sac has an inappropriate outflow for the blood that enters the sac during systole. This explanation seemed reasonable since in our study the diastolic and mean pressure

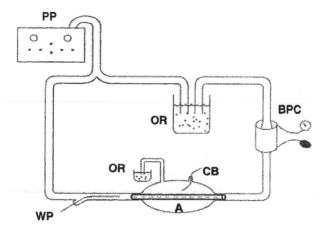

Figure 1. Diagram of ex vivo circulation: pneumatic pump (PP), aneurysm model (A), collateral branch (CB), working port (WP), blood pressure cuff (BPC), open reservoir (OR).

dropped as the outflow of the aneurysm increased. This effect can be caused by a patent collateral branch, which depressurizes the high-pressure state created by the endoleak. The effects of these residual perfusion vessels are not completely understood. The size, flow, and pressure of the outflow collateral artery in the presence of an endoleak will likely determine its ability to depressurize the aneurysm sac.

Several authors studied the effect of patent lumbar arteries as the source of endoleaks (15,16). Lumbar artery endoleaks result in some of the cases in an

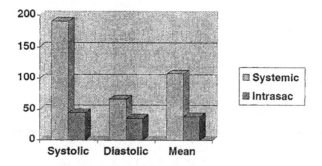

Figure 2. Systolic, diastolic, and mean pressure after the exclusion. The systemic systolic diastolic and mean pressure remained higher than the intrasac pressures.

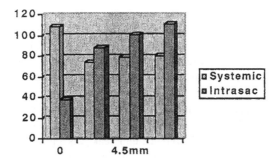

Figure 3. The mean pressure after endoleak increased significantly within the aneurysm sac and became greater than the systemic mean pressure. Similar effects on all pressure measurements were noted with larger endoleaks.

increase of the diameter of the AAA (17). Recently, Baum et al. (18) reported two techniques to measure intrasac pressures. One involves catheterization of the sac via a patent inferior mesenteric artery accessed through the superior mesenteric artery. The second, which involves direct translumbar sac puncture, is particularly promising and may facilitate effective treatment and elimination of the endoleak. They demonstrated that type II endoleaks can transmit systemic pressure to the aneurysm sac.

The behavior of AAAs treated with exclusion and bypass graft (Albany technique) facilitates our present understanding of the significance of type II endoleaks. In 1218 patients with excluded AAAs followed up for 14 years, 48 (4%) had persistent sac flow and 27 required surgery. Seven patients had rupture of their aneurysms (19).

III. TREATMENT

In our experience using the Vanguard endograft, during a mean follow-up of 28 months (range 6–48), among 100 patients, type I endoleaks were not detected. Endoleaks caused by retrograde flow from collaterals (type II endoleak) were detected in 25 cases (25%). Although retrograde collateral blood flow would appear to have a greater tendency to seal by spontaneous thrombosis, 5 patients received an additional secondary procedure because of aneurysm enlargement. Our policy is that even if they persist with associated sac shrinkage, they may be safely observed. Because of aneurysm enlargement, 5 of these patients required a secondary procedure. A limited open approach (7 cm incision) was performed in two cases, and a video-assisted clipping in the other one. In one patient a reperfusion of the aneurysmal sac via the superior mesenteric artery occurred through the inferior mesenteric artery. IMA embolization by coils was achieved via the marginal artery. In the last case the endoleak was solved by ileolumbar artery embolization.

Type III endoleaks were found in 10 cases. One patient suffered a rupture of the aneurysm after 21 months of the endoluminal treatment. His initial AAA diameter was reduced by 18 mm. A type III endoleak developed, manifested by acute back pain and CT findings corresponding to an acute aneurysm growth up to 6 cm from 3.5 cm. Cause of the type III endoleak was a graft wearing. Another patient was admitted to hospital following a syncopal episode with hypotension. A ruptured aneurysm with a limb slipped out of the main graft was diagnosed by CT scan. A surgical exploration revealed a large retroperitoneal hematoma. He died 4 days after the exploration. Another patient died due to ruptured AAA after 14 months. Details of the cause of rupture were unavailable. Complete separation of the main body from the upper two rows of the bare stent determined distal device migration with proximal endoleak, and sac repressurization was seen in 3 patients. All patients were treated by an additional proximal cuff. Component disconnection occurred in 4 patients. Distal component slipped into the sac, lying adjacent to the main body. Patients were successfully treated endoluminally placing an extension bridging the separate segments of the endograft.

We adopted the following policy to prevent endoleaks:

1. No procedure was considered finished until pressure injections of contrast media showed no type I endoleak.
2. The infra-renal aorta was covered by an endograft from the distal edge of the lower renal artery down to the iliac artery bifurcation, or to the external iliac artery if the distal common iliac or hypogastriac arteries were compromised. The device used was 20% oversized.
3. Renal artery ostia was crossed by bare stent in most of the patients and in all patients with short (1.5 cm) necks.
4. Overlapping of segments extended at least 2 cm in length.
5. Leaks from the ends were treated intraoperatively by balloon dilatation, application of cuffs, or sealed by the use of a Palmaz stent and extensions (6% of patients)
6. Gentle tension was applied to the device to prevent redundancy and consequent kinks, migration, or disengagement of segments.
7. Segments with thrombus lining the surface were not used as landing zone for the end of the device.
8. Thrombogenic materials were inserted into the aneurysm sac after the exclusion.

The decision to intervene in the presence of endoleaks depends on the size, risks, and technical possibilities. A shrinking aneurysm may be assumed to be totally depressurized. Aggressive intervention for aneurysms that are enlarging is mandatory. Although conservative management of type II endoleaks is an accepted approach, type I or III endoleaks should be repaired as soon as the diagnosis is made. With regard to aneurysm size, reduction is considered the criterion of successful treatment.

IV. ENDOTENSION

The ultimate determinant of successful AAA repair is the absence of aneurysm expansion and rupture. The expansion of aneurysms after endovascular repair is a consequence of persistent sac pressure, usually resulting from an endoleak. However, several authors have suggested that sac expansion can occur even in the absence of endoleak. This condition has been referred to by us as "pressure endoleak" and is now referred to as endotension. This entity has been associated with not only aneurysm expansion but also aneurysm rupture (20–24). Unfortunately, there is no definitive test to rule out the presence or absence of endoleak. Some authors have considered endotension as an undetected endoleak. CT scans, color duplex ultrasound (CDU) scans, and plain x-ray films were performed according to protocol to rule out any aneurysm or endograft morphological change. Angiography was occasionally performed as well, when clinically indicated. However, in some patients, despite sac enlargement, no endoleaks were detected.

The transmission of pressure through a sealed or thrombosed endoleak is one of the leading explanations for endotension if it occurs (25). If endotension results from transmission from a sealed endoleak, high-risk groups for endotension would include patients who had an endoleak that sealed spontaneously, patients in whom a migration of the endograft is seen, and patients with the endograft deployed far from the renal arteries or iliac bifurcations or on a thick layer of thrombus lining all around the aortic wall. Pressure transmission may be related to porous graft fabrics. Also, graft material has previously been responsible for the local production of serous fluid by transudation through a polytetrafluoroethylene graft used at open AAA repair (26). The mechanism for aneurysm enlargement remains unclear but is postulated to be due to pressure transmission through thrombus after endoleak thrombosis. This is correlated with the experimental demonstration that coiling with thrombosis of endoleaks fails to reduce systolic intra-aneurysmal pressures (27).

One hundred patients with AAA treated endoluminally underwent laboratory measurement of aneurysm size at baseline and at least one point in follow-up. The mean follow-up for this group was 23.2 months (range 2.0–78.8 months). The baseline major axis aneurysm size measured from 34.8 to 92.7 mm, with a mean of 57.5 ± 9.9 mm. Seventy-six were free of endoleak at all intervals and had baseline CT measurements to allow comparison. Overall, the average size decrease in this nonleaking group was 9.9 ± 9.4 mm (range − 5.6 to 11.1 mm). Evaluation for overall aneurysm expansion revealed 17 patients who had an increase of 2.3 ± 2.9 mm (range 1–11.1 mm) The only two patients with aneurysm size enlargement with no endoleak detected by CT scan were shown in plain x-ray (7.6 mm at 12 months and 11.1 mm at 36 months). Therefore, we can say that we found the explanation for every case of increase in size of the aneurysm in our series.

In the presence of nondemonstrable endoleak, no further intervention is required if the aneurysm sac is shrinking. In the presence of expansion, however, further investigation is needed to identify the source of pressurization.

Thrombosis can produce sealing of an endoleak, which may not reduce the aneurysm pressure. On other hand, intraoperative thrombosis of the sac lumen, achieved by thrombogenic material leaving into the sac, does not protect in all cases against further expansion. Lumen thrombosis does not mean pressure reduction within the aneurysm sac in which the seal of small channels in the sac is thrombotic rather than structural.

V. CONCLUSIONS

Endoleaks represent one of the main problems of the endoluminal treatment of aneurysms. Type I endoleaks can be prevented using careful techniques and are usually easily treated with cuffs or with the addition of balloon-expandable stents. Type III endoleaks represent the most serious complication of EVAR and should rapidly be resolved, preferably by endovascular techniques.

Type II endoleaks will remain a problem when all other endoleaks can be prevented. Type II endoleaks are the least dangerous of all endoleaks and are usually self-limited. They will create the same situation as with the Albany technique in which the aneurysm is isolated and the flow reestablished by a graft placed on the side of the aneurysm and anastomosed to the aorta and to the iliac arteries. A small proportion of lumbar and inferior mesenteric arteries will remain patent and produce aneurysmal growth.

Prevention of type II endoleaks can be addressed by coil embolizing the IMA and lumbar arteries or by sponge injection into the sac during the initial treatment.

Once type II endoleaks produce aneurysmal growth, they must be treated. Several treatments are possible: coil embolization of the IMA coming from the superior mesenteric artery, a laparoscopic approach, clipping of branches, embolization of the lumbar arteries from the iliolumbar branches or directly using needles and catheters placed percutaneously into the aneurysmal sac.

REFERENCES

1. May J, White GH, Waugh R, et al. Improved survival after endoluminal repair with second-generation prostheses compared with open repair in the treatment of abdominal aortic aneurysms: a 5-year concurrent comparison using life table method. J Vasc Surg 2001; 33:S21–S26.
2. Beebe HG, Cronenwett JL, Katzen BT, et al. Results of an aortic endograft trial: Impact of device failure beyond 12 months. J Vasc Surg 2001; 33:S55–S63.
3. Bush RL, Lumsden AB, Dodson TF, et al. Mid-term results after endovascular repair of the abdominal aortic aneurysm. J Vasc Surg 2001; 33:S70–S76.
4. White GH, Yu W, May J. Letter to the editors: "Endoleak"—a proposed new terminology to describe incomplete aneurysm exclusion by an endoluminal graft. J Endovasc Surg 1996; 3:124–125.
5. White GH, May J, Waugh RC. Letter to the editors: Type I and type II endoleaks: a more useful classification for reporting results of endoluminal AAA repair. J Endovasc Surg 1998; 5:189–191.
6. White GH, May J, Waugh RC. Type III and type IV endoleak: toward a complete definition of blood flow in the sac after endoluminal AAA repair. J Endovasc Surg 1998; 5:305–309.
7. Gilling-Smith GL, Cuypers P, Buth J. The significance of endoleaks after endovascular aneurysm repair: results of a large European multicenter study (abstr). J Endovasc Surg 1998; 5:1–12.
8. Chuter TAM, Ivancev K, Malina M. Aneurysm pressure following endovascular exclusion. Eur J Vasc Endovasc Surg 1997; 13:85–87.
9. May J, White GH, Yu W. A prospective study of changes in morphology and dimensions of abdominal aortic aneurysms following endoluminal repair: a preliminary report. J Endovasc Surg 1995; 2:343–347.
10. Matsumura JS, Pearce WH, McCarthy WJ. Reduction in aortic aneurysm size: early results after endovascular graft placement. J Vasc Surg 1997; 25:113–123.
11. Parodi JC. Endovascular repair of abdominal aortic aneurysms and other arterial lesions. J Vasc Surg 1995; 21:549–557.
12. Lumsden AB, Allen RC, Chaikof EL. Delayed rupture of aortic aneurysms following endovascular stent grafting. Am J Surg 1995; 170:174–178.

13. White GH, Yu W, May J. Three-year experience with the White-Yu Endovascular-GAD Graft for transluminal repair of aortic and iliac aneurysms. J Endovasc Surg 1997; 4:124–136.

14. Resch T, Ivancev K, Lindh M. Persistent collateral perfusion of abdominal aortic aneurysm after endovascular repair does not lead to progressive change in aneurysm diameter. J Vasc Surg 1998; 28:242–249.

15. Singh-Ranger R, McArthur T, Raphael M. What happens to abdominal aortic aneurysms after endovascular grafting? A volumetric study using spiral CT angiography. J Intervent Radiol 1998; 13:145–146.

16. Liewald F, Ermis C, et al. Influence of treatment of type II leaks on the aneurysm surface area. Eur J Vasc Endovasc Surg 2001; 21(4):339–343.

17. Gilling-Smith GL, Martin J, Sudhindran S, et al. Freedom from endoleak after endovascular aneurysm repair does not equal treatment success. Eur J Vasc Endovasc Surg 2000; 19(4):421–425.

18. Baum RA, Carpenter JP, Cope C, Golden MA, Velazquez OC, Neschis DG, Mitchell ME, Barker CF, Fairman RM. Aneurysm sac pressure measurements after endovascular repair of abdominal aortic aneurysms. J Vasc Surg 2001; 33(1):32–41.

19. Resnikoff M, Clement Darling R III, Chang BB, Lloyd WE, Paty PSK, Leather RP, Shah DM. Fate of the excluded abdominal aortic aneurysm sac: long-term follow-up of 831 patients. J Vasc Surg 1996; 24(5):851–855.

20. White GH, May J. How should endotension be defined? History of a concept and evolution of a new term. J Endovasc Ther 2000; 7(6):435–438.

21. White GH, May J, Petrasek P, et al. Endotension: an explanation for continued AAA growth after successful endoluminal repair. J Endovasc Surg 1999; 6(4):308–315.

22. Gilling-Smith G, Brennan J, Harris P. Endotension after endovascular aneurysm repair: definition, classification, and strategies for surveillance and intervention. J Endovasc Surg 1999; 6(4):305–307.

23. Meier GH, Parker FM, et al. Endotension after endovascular aneurysm repair: the Ancure experience. J Vasc Surg 2001; 34(3):421–427.

24. Bade MA, Ohki T, et al. Hypogastric artery aneurysm rupture after endovascular graft exclusion with shrinkage of the aneurysm: significance of endotension from a "virtual," or thrombosed type II endoleak. J Vasc Surg 2001; 33(6):1271–1274.

25. Ruurda JP, Rijbroek A, et al. Continuing expansion of internal iliac artery aneurysms after surgical exclusion of the inflow. A report of two cases. J Cardiovasc Surg (Torino) 2001; 42(3):389–392.

26. Williams GM. The management of massive ultrafiltration distending the aneurysm sac after abdominal aortic aneurysm repair with a polytetrafluoro-ethylene aortobi-iliac graft. J Vasc Surg 1998; 28:551–555.

27. Marty B, Sanchez LA, Ohki T. Endoleak after endovascular graft repair of experimental aortic aneurysms: Does coil embolization with angiographic "seal" lower intra-aneurysmal pressure? J Vasc Surg 1998; 27:454–462.

9

The Nature and Significance of Endoleak and Endotension: The Liverpool View

Geoffrey L. Gilling-Smith and Peter Lyon Harris
University of Liverpool and Royal Liverpool University Hospital, Liverpool, England

I. DEFINITIONS

An endoleak is defined as blood flow within the aneurysm sac but outside the stent graft following endovascular repair (1,2). Endoleaks are classified according to their sites of origin (Table 1). Endotension* is defined as persistent or recurrent pressurization of the aneurysm sac following endovascular repair (3). Endotension is classified into three grades according to its association with blood flow within the aneurysm sac (Table 2).

Both endoleak and endotension are evidence of failure to isolate the aneurysm sac from the circulation. In every other respect, however, these two phenomena, although often related, are quite different.

The diagnosis of endoleak relies on the observation of contrast medium within the aneurysm sac on angiography, computed tomography (CT), or Duplex scanning. We conclude from such an observation that blood is able to flow into the aneurysm sac and we may be able to discern the route by which it

---

*Endotension—literally tension within. The word tension was chosen because of its dual meaning. In English it describes the force acting on the aneurysm wall. It is also the French word for blood pressure.

Table 1.   Classification of Endoleaks

Type of endoleak	Intrasac flow	Possible intervention
I	Perigraft flow at proximal or distal graft attachment site	Cuff/extension Conversion
II	Flow through side branches (e.g., lumbar, IMA)	Coil embolization Laparoscopic or open ligation Conservative
III	Fabric tear or modular disconnection	Covered stent Secondary endograft Conversion
IV	Graft porosity	Conservative

does so. What we cannot assess simply from the observation of an endoleak is the pressure that may or may not be associated with flow of blood. Nor can we, with any certainty, determine the magnitude of hemorrhage that might occur should the aneurysm rupture.

Endotension, on the other hand, cannot be observed. Endotension or intrasac pressure is a force that acts on the aneurysm wall and may cause the aneurysm to expand and/or rupture. It should be noted, however, that the aneurysm may not, in fact, expand or rupture and that the diagnosis of endotension cannot be excluded merely because the aneurysm fails to expand.

A useful analogy is provided by the concept of gravity. This describes the force that acts upon an object, such as an apple, and that may cause it to fall to the ground. The apple may not fall if it is securely tethered to the branch of the tree, but it would be nonsense to suggest that gravity did not exist simply because the apple did not fall to the ground.

It should also be noted that expansion of an aneurysm is not necessarily evidence of pressure. It is quite conceivable that an aneurysm can continue to expand as a result of continued accumulation of fluid or other material without

Table 2.   Classification of Endotension

Grade	Intrasac pressure	Intrasac flow (potential for hemorrhage)
I	High	High (e.g., graft-related endoleak)
II	High	Low (e.g., side branch endoleak)
III	High	Absent

such accumulation resulting in pressurization of the aneurysm. Thus the diagnosis of endotension relies on accurate measurement of intrasac pressure.

II. CLINICAL SIGNIFICANCE

The risk of aneurysm rupture depends primarily on the size of the aneurysm, the pressure within it, and the force applied to the aneurysm wall. The clinical consequence of rupture, however, depends primarily on the potential for life-threatening hemorrhage, and this, in turn, depends on the rate at which blood can flow into and then out of the aneurysm once rupture has occurred. In order to assess the clinical significance of endoleak or endotension, therefore, one must evaluate the risk of aneurysm rupture and the risk of life-threatening hemorrhage should rupture occur.

A. Graft-Related Endoleak

There is general agreement (and it is almost certainly true) that graft-related endoleaks transmit systemic pressure to the aneurysm sac. If the aneurysm is large, the risk of rupture is probably significant, although it should be noted that the relationship between pressure and rupture is not well understood. We do not, for example, know what pressure is required to cause an aneurysm to rupture, nor do we know whether it matters if the pressure is constant (i.e., no pulse pressure) or varies throughout the cardiac cycle.

It is highly likely that in most cases the flow of blood through a graft-related endoleak would be sufficient to cause a major clinical problem should rupture occur. Hemorrhage may well be less catastrophic than that which occurs following rupture of an untreated aneurysm, but it is, in most cases, likely to be sufficient to cause acute hemodynamic instability. There are now many anecdotal reports of rupture and death in association with untreated graft-related endoleak. In the absence of any hard evidence to the contrary (and it would probably now be unethical to conduct any form of trial to obtain such evidence), we believe that all graft-related endoleaks present a serious threat to the patient.

B. Side Branch Endoleak

The clinical significance of side branch endoleak, on the other hand, remains very uncertain. There have been conflicting reports of both high and low intrasac pressure in association with such endoleaks. There have also been reports of both aneurysm shrinkage and aneurysm rupture in the presence of type II endoleak.

We believe (and have anecdotal evidence from our own practice) that some side branch endoleaks cause significant pressurization of the aneurysm sac, while others do not. The question, therefore, is whether the risk of hemorrhage is significant should rupture occur as a result of a type II endoleak. Again, we do not know. It is probable, however, that the risk of fatal hemorrhage is very much less than with graft-related endoleak.

C. Endotension

Since it is intrasac pressure that causes expansion and ultimately rupture of an aneurysm, it follows that an aneurysm that remains or is again pressurized is at risk of rupture, the magnitude of that risk depending on the size of the aneurysm as well as the nature and severity of intrasac pressure. Thus, if endotension is present, the patient is at risk.

The consequences of such rupture depend on the cause of endotension. If it is due to a graft-related endoleak, the potential for hemorrhage is significant (see above). If it is associated with low-flow type II endoleak, the potential for hemorrhage much less (hence the rationale for classifying endotension according to the potential for hemorrhage). But what if the aneurysm is pressurized through thrombus or microleaks? Could it not be argued that rupture might have no clinical consequence at all?

The consequence of rupture in the absence of endoleak is difficult to predict. To a certain extent the outcome of such an event depends on the security of fixation of the endograft. If the aneurysm is pressurized but has not expanded and if there is no evidence of migration, then rupture is likely to be a relatively benign event. If, on the other hand, endotension has resulted in expansion of the aneurysm, it may well have resulted in expansion and/or shortening of the aneurysm neck so that the security of endograft fixation is compromised. Untreated, such expansion might result in secondary graft-related endoleak, rupture, and significant hemorrhage. In general, therefore, we consider endotension in the absence of endoleak to be significant if there is measurable expansion of the aneurysm and/or a significant change in the geometry of the aneurysm.

III. SURVEILLANCE AFTER ENDOVASCULAR REPAIR

Our surveillance protocol is based on serial clinical and radiological examination of the patient. Detailed discussion of the relative merits of different imaging modalities is beyond the scope of this chapter, but like many centers we continue to rely on CT scanning as the backbone of our surveillance protocol. Scans are reviewed both for evidence of endoleak and for evidence of aneurysm enlargement. Angiography is employed selectively to define the source of endoleak where this is uncertain. Translumbar sac pressure measurement is employed selectively in patients with large aneurysms that fail to shrink and in patients with aneurysms that are expanding where the cause for this is uncertain.

IV. INDICATIONS FOR SECONDARY INTERVENTION

Secondary endovascular or open surgical intervention should, in our view, be considered if there is evidence that the patient remains or is again at risk from aneurysm rupture. The decision to intervene depends, in the final analysis, on the perceived balance of risks. In each case one must evaluate the risks of any proposed intervention and balance these against the risk of rupture and hemorrhage. Unfortunately this is rarely straightforward. Only limited data are available about the risks of secondary intervention, and it is in any case difficult to quantify the risk in any individual patient. In many cases it is also very difficult to predict the likelihood of rupture and hemorrhage, so that the decision to intervene or not is more often than not based on instinct, intuition, or gut feeling—art rather than science. It seems to us that we have as a result tended to overreact and perhaps intervene excessively and unnecessarily.

In general, we advocate intervention to deal with any documented graft-related endoleak. Such leaks can usually be treated by secondary endovascular intervention (i.e., by endovascular placement of a cuff or graft limb extension). Should an endovascular approach fail, however, one may have to consider conversion to conventional repair. This is a relatively high-risk intervention with reported major morbidity and mortality in excess of 20%. The operative risk may well be greater than the risk of death from aneurysm rupture, and the decision to proceed to conversion is not, therefore, straightforward.

We have, over the last few years, become more conservative in our approach to side branch endoleaks. These can often be treated by coil embolization or by laparoscopic clipping, but both techniques are associated with risks, and we have started to question whether or not such risks are justified. More often than not we will simply observe patients with type II endoleaks, monitoring the morphology of the aneurysm and, in particular, the aneurysm neck. We will not, in general, intervene unless the aneurysm is very large, expanding rapidly, and/or associated with evidence of graft migration.

We routinely measure intrasac pressure in patients with large aneurysms that are not shrinking, in patients with expanding aneurysms where the cause of expansion is uncertain, and in patients with evidence of side branch endoleak of uncertain significance. The problem with intrasac pressure measurement is that we do not always know what the result means. If the pressure within the aneurysm sac is no greater than surrounding tissue pressure, one may conclude that the aneurysm has been isolated from the circulation and that the risk of rupture is negligible. This assumes of course that the measurement obtained is accurate and reflects the pressure throughout the aneurysm sac (which may or may not be the case).

If, on the other hand, the pressure within the aneurysm sac is elevated, one may conclude that the aneurysm is not isolated from the circulation and in theory at least remains at risk of rupture. It is, however, very difficult to know whether this risk is significant, particularly if the pressure within the sac is less than systemic pressure and/or nonpulsatile. This is important since in the absence of endoleak the only therapeutic option is conversion to open repair, a procedure that may well submit the patient to greater risk than continued observation.

V. SUMMARY

Endoleak describes flow within the excluded aneurysm sac.

Endotension describes pressure within the excluded aneurysm sac.

Endoleak is clinically significant if associated with significant intrasac pressure.

Endotension is clinically significant if associated with the potential for hemorrhage in the event of aneurysm rupture or if it causes progressive enlargement of the aneurysm and aneurysm neck so that the security of endograft fixation is compromised.

It is not known what pressure within the aneurysm sac is necessary to cause rupture, nor is it known whether or not a pulsatile wave form is more dangerous than a flat one.

REFERENCES

1.   White GH, May J, Waugh RC, Yu W. MS type I and type II endoleaks: a more useful classification for reporting results of endoluminal AAA repair. J Endovasc Surg 1998; 5:189–193.

2. White GH, May J, Waugh RC, Chaufour X, Yu W. Type III and type IV endoleak: toward a complete definition of blood flow in the sac after endoluminal AAA repair. J Endovasc Surg 1998; 5:305–309.
3. Gilling-Smith G, Brennan J, Harris P, Bakran A, Gould D, McWilliams R. Endotension after endovascular aneurysm repair: definition, classification, and strategies for surveillance and intervention. J Endovasc Surg 1999; 6:305–307.

10

AAA Endograft Endoleak Management

Rodney A. White, Irwin Walot, and Carlos Donayre
Harbor-UCLA Medical Center, Torrance, California, U.S.A.

I. INTRODUCTION

As endovascular prostheses have been developed to exclude abdominal aortic aneurysms (AAAs), new concepts related to the selection and surveillance of patients have evolved. Endoleaks and endotension are phenomena that were not initially anticipated but that now are of great interest in the effort to understand the etiology and implications of leaks and to identify patients requiring intervention to obliterate leaks.

The following discussion describes our current approach to the identification, surveillance, and treatment of endoleaks as it has evolved in our clinical practice over the last several years. Our current perspectives are based on particular patient scenarios that have occurred and represent an ongoing assessment of appropriate therapy.

II. DEFINITIONS

The definition of an endoleak for this discussion will be evidence of blood flow in the aneurysm sac after attempted exclusion with an endovascular prosthesis. Evidence of blood flow may be by contrast enhancement on angiography or computed tomography (CT) or flow-visualized by duplex ultrasound or magnetic resonance angiography.

Endoleaks are classified by time of occurrence as follows:

Acute—at the time of the procedure or following the procedure within the first 30 days

Persistent—from the time of the procedure and continuing longer than 30 days

Late—beginning at some interval following the procedure

Leaks are also categorized by the origin of the endoleak:

Proximal or distal attachment site (type I)

Junctional—at the connection of modular components (type I)

Collateral flow—filling of the aneurysm from branch arteries, i.e., lumbar, mesenteric, accessory renal, etc. (type II)

Graft—related to fabric porosity, suture holes, or material defects

This classification system is compatible with systems that have been described by other investigators (1,2).

III. ASSUMPTIONS AND OBSERVATIONS

As with any discussion regarding endoleaks, it must be stated that the implication of leaks is unknown. The assumption that pressurized leaks, i.e., communications between the blood flow and the aneurysm wall that transmit arterial pressure, can lead to rupture is supported by knowledge of the pathophysiology of aneurysms. For this reason, proximal, distal, or large junctional type I leaks should be treated as soon as possible in order to accomplish the primary goal of exclusion of the aneurysm. Although this type of leak has been reported to seal in a percentage of patients over time, the thrombus seal that is accomplished in many cases may still transmit arterial pressure and thus not effectively exclude the aneurysm. "Endotension" or pressurization of the aneurysm sac that persists following apparent endograft exclusion is developing as a concept that may explain persistent pressurization when there is no enhancement of the aneurysm during contrast studies.

Other types of endoleaks, such as transgraft flow or filling of the aneurysm via patent collaterals with no communication to the blood vessel lumen or the body of the endograft (type II), present more difficult diagnostic problems. In many patients there are numerous collateral vessels that fill the aneurysm that are visualized at the time of diagnostic CT or conventional angiography preintervention that have unknown potential for continued or late collateral filling of the aneurysm. In many patients there may be evidence of diffuse collateralization at the time of the procedure with most of the vessels thrombosing over a short interval following exclusion. There are a few patients that have collaterals that fill the aneurysm and that persist for a significant time following the procedure. There is also an additional group of patients with collateral filling of the aneurysm that begins at some interval following the procedure and which increases in flow and size with time.

IV. OUR ALGORITHM FOR ENDOLEAK MANAGEMENT

There have been various approaches to the collaterals that fill the aneurysm sac after endovascular repair. Aggressive initial identification and embolization represents the approach that appears to have little benefit, particularly because of significant complications related to the embolization procedure (3). An exception to this observation is the large accessory renal arteries that arise from the aneurysm. We reported a late aneurysm rupture from a lumbar-asessory renal artery endoleak in a patient who declined intervention to thrombose this vessel (4). Observation of the collaterals to eliminate those that spontaneously thrombose is the most frequent approach. This method is appealing because many of the collateral connections eventually occlude. Some of the late-appearing collateral channels appear and then thrombose with no apparent implication on aneurysm decompression. The remaining collateral pathways follow an unpredictable course, with continued observation being the current method to determine the need for intervention. The most puzzling group of collateral reperfusions are the leaks that appear late, persist and enlarge with obvious pressurization of the aneurysm.

We believe that once a collateral channel is found to persistently fill the aneurysm, there must be an outlet channel that permits continuing flow. If the source of inflow or outflow is the endoluminal prosthesis, than the potential for pressurization is significant and this type of endoleak should be treated. The assessment for need for intervention in other types of endoleaks is less clear and in our institution is based upon the well-established understanding that the risk of aneurysm rupture is directly associated with the size of the aneurysm and an increasing diameter. For this reason, our criteria for intervention are based on serial imaging that permits quantitation of aneurysm diameter, volume, and morphology in addition to an assessment of endoleak flow. Using this approach, we have observed a number of patients with collateral endoleaks and persistent flow with no evidence for aneurysm diameter or volume increase, and no change in morphology that is concerning (5). In other cases we have intervened when morphology changes might eventually lead to development of a pressurized leak even when volumes and diameters were stable or decreasing. Current evidence suggests that all endoleaks are pressurized, i.e., can be measured to have significant pressure approximating systemic arterial pressure (6).

Although this observation has been substantiated by many investigators, most type II leaks do not appear to pressurize the entire aneurysm beyond the local perfusion site because the aneurysms do not increase in size and may decrease over time.

In the situation where a collateral endoleak is identified, careful analysis of spiral CT reconstructions is performed to identify the source of the leak. If this is not possible or if there is evidence of aneurysm enlargement, arteriographic assessment of the aneurysm is performed. Based on the combination of angiographic findings and the morphological data acquired from the spiral three-dimensional (3-D) CT analysis, the aneurysms may be observed or an intervention with injection of thrombotic substances into the aneurysm sac and selective collateral vessel embolization planned (7). In a situation where persistent collateralization remains following interventions that do not prevent enlargement, conversion to open surgical repair is then considered (8).

In our practice we carefully follow patients for localized or overall aneurysm enlargement due to leaks with the current algorithm developed to address several issues. We have also increased surveillance of patients with aneurysms that do not decrease in size after 12–18 months to observe for potential sources of entension even if endoleaks are not apparent on contrast studies (5).

V. OUR CURRENT SURVEILLANCE PROTOCOL

Patients for endografts are chosen for the procedure based on spiral contrast CT imaging and 3-D reconstructions prepared by a member of the team that is intimately familiar with the patient selection criterion and device specifications. Careful documentation of aneurysm morphology based on MIPS (maximal intensity projection) curvalinear reconstructions to assess the degree of vascular wall calcifications, tortuousity, and device length requirements. Fixation site diameters are measured on axial slices displayed perpendicular to the centerline of the vessel lumen to prevent measurement errors due to data averaging on thicker slice axial images or from angulation artifacts produced on axial images displayed perpendicular to the long axis of the patient. Ancillary studies including preintervention angiography or IVUS imaging are used only when required to clarify issues not addressed by the CT. Although the preintervention imaging protocol is not frequently considered as part of the surveillance data, it is particularly important that this information be carefully acquired and stored for later reference so that subsequent studies can be carefully interpreted in conjunction with the preintervention data. In many cases, conventional film storage of patient data is space and time consuming for busy interventional services, and the development of cost-efficient, automated methods to store patient data and images is a priority for current development that is being addressed in prototype studies (5).

Our postprocedure imaging protocol consists of imaging the device with 30 days with contrast CT to assure firm fixation and evaluate endoleak status. If there are any concerns regarding aneurysm exclusion at the conclusion of the procedure, a contrast CT is performed prior to patient discharge. In most cases, the postprocedure CT is delayed for 30 days to allow for sealing and avoid visualization of early contrast enhancement which can occur due to transgraft flow in porous fabric devices or due to flow via collaterals that seal shortly following the procedure. The CT contrast protocols always include a precontrast CT acquired at 5 mm intervals to document the patterns of vascular calcification, followed by a spiral contrast CT acquired at 2–3 mm intervals with 3-D reconstructions prepared using the methodology described previously. A postprocedure non-contrast 5 mm interval scan is also acquired 8–12 minutes following the contrast study to assess late aneurysm enhancement. Post procedure duplex color assessment of the device and/or multiple isomorphous replacement angiography are used to assess the device if contrast is contraindicated (9).

If the aneurysm is excluded at 30 days with no contrast enhancement, follow-up evaluations are performed at 6 months, 1 year, and then yearly to evaluate aneurysm morphology and exclusion. Interactive CT reconstructions using software specifically designed to assess aneurysm and device morphology have enhanced surveillance accuracy and identification of indications for secondary interventions (5).

In patients with aneurysm enhancement, angiography is needed to clearly identify the etiology of the endoleak. If a type I leak is identified, secondary interventions are performed expeditiously to assure depressurization of the aneurysm. If aneurysm enhancement is via the inferior mesenteric artery (IMA) or lumbar vessels, repeat CT is performed at 3 months to observe progression of the endoleak volume, aneurysm diameter, and aneurysm volume. If no change is seen at 3 months, repeat imaging at 3-month intervals is performed to observe progression. Based on our experience with increased aneurysm size over time related to either lumbar to IMA or accessory renal artery circuits (4,5,8), intervention to thrombose the aneurysm by combined injection of the thrombotic substances into the aneurysm sac plus selective coil occlusion of branch vessels is attempted if the endoleaks persist beyond 6–12 months (Figs. 1 and 2). This approach has led to aneurysm thrombosis and prevention of aneurysm enlargement in most cases, although repeated coil embolizations are occasionally required (7).

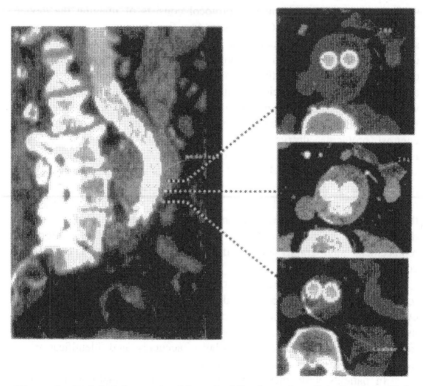

Figure 1. Endoleak that persisted 6 months following endograft deployment with the lumbar-IMA pathway identifiable by computer 3-D image analysis. This type of endoleak is observed with increased surveillance, including volumes, with evidence of endoleak or aneurysm enlargement or persistence beyond one year leading to a recommendation for thrombotic injection of the endoleak and coil embolization of the IMA.

Pre-Procedure   **1 Year Post-Deployment**

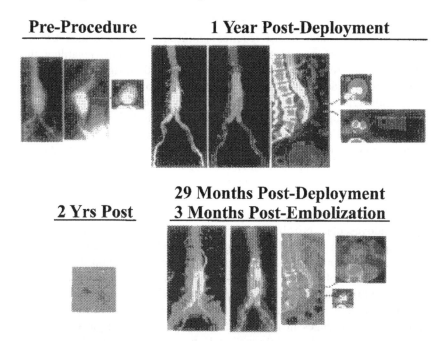

2 Yrs Post   **29 Months Post-Deployment**
                    3 Months Post-Embolization

Figure 2.   Endoleak of lumbar origin that persisted for 2 years following endograft deployment with increase in aneurysm diameter (3 mm) and volume (180–190 cc). Coil embolization and thrombin injection at 2 years resolved leak on 3-month follow-up after the second intervention.

VI. ENDOGRAFT SURVEILLANCE—A MANDATORY COMPONENT FOR LONG-TERM SUCCESS

Surveillance of endovascular devices used to treat aortic aneurysms is needed to assess the function of the device, to observe accommodation of the device to morphological changes of the aneurysm, and to determine the need for intervention for new phenomena that have been identified, such as endoleaks. Surveillance of endografts presents a new challenge because conventional surgical procedures require no routine imaging for follow-up, with current assessment being limited to physical examination, including pulses and ankle-brachial indices. Imaging studies are only used when conventional repairs are compromised by recurrence of lesions, infections, or other complications. Surveillance images must be interpreted expediously with results readily available for patient encounters and clinical decisions. Not only does this require significant increase in time for repetitive office visits and interpretation of studies, it also requires significant resources to store data for later reference. At present there are unanswered questions regarding the reimbursement for these services provided by both imaging centers and physicians that add a new dimension to the adaptation of this technology.

Although many imaging modalities can be used to choose patients and perform follow-up evaluations following endograft deployment, the most widely used and readily accessible technology is contrast CT scanning. In many centers performing complex aneurysm repairs, spiral (helical) CT reconstructions are being used with increasing frequency. New algorithms that permit analysis of the CT data in an interactive environment provide a means to perform needed evaluations (5).

As centers accumulate larger numbers of patients who have been treated with endovascular prostheses, the volume of CT examinations and information being collected can overcome individual physician capabilities to perform comprehensive surveillance. A recently developed algorithm utilizes transfer of the CT data to a central laboratory that performs the interactive function and reports on important surveillance phenomena such as integrity of the aneurysm, endoleaks, aneurysm size (volume), and morphological changes in the device related to morphological changes of the aneurysm. This basic information is then transferred to the patient's electronic record. In this way, rapid and accurate availability of the patient record and imaging for physician assessment and patient encounters minimizes the time and effort required to coordinate this essential assessment.

At present, several investigators are investigating the utility of electronic record analysis as a means to enhance appropriate patient selection and increase the efficiency of postimplant surveillance. Other innovative means to perform the same function may also evolve as more physicians become focused on resolving this need in an expedient manner.

REFERENCES

1. White GH, Yu Weiyun, May J. "Endoleak"—a proposed new terminology to describe incomplete aneurysm exclusion by an endoluminal graft. J Endovasc Surg 1996; 3:123–125.
2. Beebe HG. Leaks after endovascular therapy for aneurysm: detection and classification. J Endovasc Surg 1996; 3:445–448.
3. Resch T, Ivancer K, Lindh M, Ulfn, Brunkwall J, Molina M, Lindblad B. Persistent collateral perfusion of abdominal aortic aneurysm after endovascular repair does

not lead to progressive change in aneurysm diameter. J Vasc Surg 1998; 28:242–249.

4. White RA, Donayre CE, Walot I, Stewart M. Abdominal aortic aneurysm rupture following endograft repair: report of a predictable event. J Endovasc Ther 2000; 7:257–262.

5. White RA, Donayre CE, Walot I, Woody J, Kim N, Kopchok GE. Computed tomography assessment of abdominal aortic aneurysm morphology after endograft exclusion. J Vasc Surg 2001; 31:S1–10.

6. Baum RA, Carpenter JP, Cope C, Golden M, Vasquez O, Neschis DG, et al. Aneurysm sac pressure measurements after endovascular repair of abdominal aortic aneurysms. J Vasc Surg 2001; 33:32–41.

7. Walot I, White RA, Donayre CE, Soto CF. Treatment of endoleaks following abdominal aortic stent grafting. Techniques and volumetric analysis to determine indications and assess outcomes. J Vasc and Interventional Radiology 2001; 12(suppl):5120.

8. White RA, Walot I, Donayre CE, Woody J, Kopchok GE. Failed AAA endograft exclusion due to type II endoleak: explant analysis. J Endovasc Ther 2001; 8:254–261.

9. Wolf Y, Johnson B, Hill B, Rubin B, Fogarty T, Zerins C. Duplex ultrasound scanning versus computer tomographic angiography for post operative evaluation of endovascular aortic aneurysm. J Vasc Surg 2000; 32:1142–1148.

11

Endoleaks Do Not Predict Clinical Outcome Following Endovascular Aneurysm Repair

Christopher K. Zarins
Stanford University, Stanford, California, U.S.A.

I. INTRODUCTION

Endoleak is considered by many to be evidence of treatment failure of endovascular aneurysm repair and has been called "the major complication of endovascular aneurysm repair" (1–3). However, it is not clear that endoleak in and of itself represents an adverse event of the procedure. Rather, endoleak is simply radiographic or ultrasonic evidence of continued blood flow in the aneurysm sac following placement of an endovascular stent graft. Since the primary objective of any treatment of aortic aneurysms is to prevent rupture and death from rupture, we sought to determine whether the presence or absence of endoleak following endovascular repair is a determinant or predictor of subsequent clinical outcome. We compared patients with and without endoleak as determined by postprocedure contrast computed tomography (CT) scan with respect to three primary outcome measures— death, aneurysm rupture, and conversion to open surgical repair—and found that the presence or absence of endoleak does not predict the major adverse clinical events following endovascular repair (4).

II. STUDY DESIGN

All patients treated during Phase II of the multicenter clinical trial of endovascular aneurysm repair using the Medtronic AneuRx stent graft system (5) were reviewed. Full data sets and selected cross-sectional images of noncontrast and contrast infused spiral CT scans performed prior to hospital discharge were evaluated by the investigators at each of the 13 study sites (centers) and reported to the AneuRx Clinical Data Base. Selected cross-sectional images of the predischarge CT along with abdominal x-rays were sent for blinded reading to an independent radiology group (core lab), which had no involvement with any of the clinical investigation sites. A total of 398 patients had successful implantations of the stent graft and had a predischarge CT image available for analysis by the centers. Of these, 350 were evaluated by the core lab.

Patients were grouped according to whether or not an endoleak was present and separate analyses were performed based on endoleak status as defined by the centers or by the core lab.

III. ENDOLEAK RATE

The endoleak rate prior to hospital discharge was 38% as reported by the centers and 50% as reported by the core lab ($p < 0.001$). Endoleaks were classified as type I (device related) in 30%, type II (branch flow) in 40%, and undetermined in 30%. The higher endoleak rate reported by the core lab persisted at 6 months and one year. The endoleak rate reported from the centers was 16% at 6 months and 13% at one year compared to an endoleak rate of 27% at 6 months and 20% at one year reported by the core lab ($p < 0.001$). However, there was no difference in the rate of detection of new endoleaks (6%), stent graft migration (2%), or aneurysm enlargement (6%) between the centers and core lab readings.

IV. PRIMARY OUTCOME MEASURES

Twenty patients have died during the follow-up period. No patient died of aneurysm rupture. There was no difference in mortality rate for patients with endoleak (5%) on predischarge CT compared to patients without endoleak (5%). There was no difference in mortality rate between center- and core lab–defined endoleak.

One patient had aneurysm rupture during the study period. This patient had a minor endoleak on CT scan one day after successful placement of the stent graft by both center and core lab reading. One month later neither the center nor the core lab reported an endoleak and aneurysm size was unchanged. At 6 and 12 months there was no endoleak and no change in aneurysm size. Two months later the patient experienced back pain and a CT scan demonstrated rupture of the aneurysm.

Two patients (0.5%) underwent successful open surgical repair (surgical conversion) during the follow-up period. One was the patient with rupture described above. A second patient had endoleak at discharge, 1 month, and 6 months due to a proximal type I endoleak with no change in aneurysm size. The patient declined a recommendation to place a proximal extender cuff and chose to undergo elective open surgical repair.

V. NEW ENDOLEAKS

A new endoleak during the course of the study was documented by the centers in 9% of patients and by the core lab in 6% of patients. There was no difference in the appearance rate of new endoleaks between patients with or without endoleak at hospital discharge as determined by the centers or the core lab. There was no difference in new endoleak between patients with or without endoleak at one month. Among the 32 patients with new onset endoleak identified by the centers, six (19%) had an additional procedure that successfully treated the endoleak; three of these new endoleaks were related to stent graft migration.

VI. OUTCOME BY ENDOLEAK TYPE

Outcome by endoleak type was determined by the core laboratory. There were no differences in death from any cause or aneurysm rupture rate between patients with type I or type II endoleaks and those with no endoleaks. Patients with type I endoleaks were more likely to undergo surgical conversion and experience aneurysm enlargement compared with patients with no type I endoleak ($p < 0.05$). Patients with type II endoleak were less likely to experience a new endoleak compared with patients without type II endoleaks ($p = 0.05$).

VII. PRIMARY OUTCOME SUCCESS

Since the primary objective of aortic aneurysm repair is to prevent aneurysm rupture and death from rupture, we considered a successful primary outcome following endovascular aneurysm repair to be rupture-free survival with a patent stent-graft and no need for an additional procedure or conversion to open surgical repair. A successful primary outcome following stent-graft repair, by Kaplan-Meier analysis, was achieved in 92% of patients at 12 months and 88% of patients at 18 months in this study. There was no significant difference in primary outcome between patients with and those without endoleak at the time of hospital discharge. This was true whether the center or core lab determination of endoleak was used for the analysis.

Rupture-free survival with a patent graft and no conversion to open surgical repair was achieved by utilizing additional procedures to treat endoleak or nonpatency of the graft in 6% of patients. This resulted in a secondary outcome success of 96% at 12 months and 94% at 18 months. There was no difference is secondary outcome between patients with and those without endoleak at the time of hospital discharge. This was true whether the center or core lab determination was used for the analysis.

VIII. DISCUSSION

Our results show that endoleak at hospital discharge is not a predictor of primary or secondary outcome following endovascular aneurysm repair. Nor is endoleak at discharge a predictor of aneurysm enlargement, stent-graft patency, stent-graft migration, or the appearance of new endoleaks. We compared endoleak as evaluated by individual study sites to endoleak evaluated independently and in a blinded manner by a central core laboratory. There was a significant difference in endoleak rate as evaluated by the study sites and by the core laboratory based on evaluation of the same contrast infused CT scans. However, the centers had the advantage of the complete data set of spiral CT images with both pre- and postcontrast infusion images as well as delayed images, while the core lab may not always have had the noncontrast CT images to help differentiate calcium from contrast in the aneurysm sac. Thus, the higher reading of endoleak in the core lab may be due, in part, to interpretation of calcium as endoleak. This highlights the difficulty in using the interpretation of endoleak with precision. Nonetheless, there was no difference in evaluation of clinically significant features such as the appearance of a new endoleak, change in aneurysm size, or evidence of stent-graft migration between study sites and the core lab. Furthermore, there was no difference in outcome analysis regardless of whether the centers or core lab assessment of endoleak was used.

A number of investigators have focused on endoleak, identifying it as the primary failure mode of endovascular repair, and closely related it to risk of aneurysm rupture (1–3). However, many reports include a variety of stent grafts of varying design, many in the early stages of development (1,2), making it difficult to evaluate the true overall outcome of endovascular repair. Many of the ruptures and failures have been related to fabric or device structural failure (6–10), which may not occur in improved stent graft designs. While failures have been linked to endoleaks, endoleak may simply be the method by which the failure was identified and demonstrated, rather than providing evidence that flow in the aneurysm sac is the prerequisite cause of rupture (11).

In conclusion, endoleak is commonly seen following endovascular repair but is a poor predictor of subsequent outcome event. Thus, the focus on endoleak as a primary outcome measure of endovascular aneurysm repair may be unfounded. While it is important to carefully monitor all patients with endovascular grafts, absence of endoleak or the prevention of or treatment of endoleak should not defocus attention from the more important considerations of aneurysm size and patient clinical status.

REFERENCES

1. Harris PL. The highs and lows of endovascular aneurysm repair: the first two years of the Eurostar Registry. Ann R Coll Surg Engl 1999; 81:161–165.
2. Schurink GWH, Aarts NJM, van Bockel JH. Endoleak after stent-graft treatment of abdominal aortic aneurysm: a meta-analysis of clinical studies. Br J Surg 1999; 86:581–587.
3. White GH, Yu W, May J, Chaufour X, Stephen MS. Endoleak as a complication of endoluminal grafting of abdominal aortic aneurysms: classification, incidence, diagnosis, and management. J Endovasc Surg 1997; 4:152–168.
4. Zarins CK, White RA, Hodgson KJ, Schwarten D, Fogarty TJ. Endoleak as a predictor of outcome after endovascular aneurysm repair: AneuRx multicenter clinical trial. J Vasc Surg 2000; 32:90–107.
5. Zarins CK, White RA, Schwarten D, Kinney K, Diethrich EB, Hodgson KH, Fogarty TJ. for the Investigators of the Medtronic AneuRx Multicenter Clinical Trial. AneuRx stent graft vs. open surgical repair of abdominal aortic aneurysms: Multicenter Prospective Clinical Trial. J Vasc Surg 1999; 29:292–308.
6. White GH, May J, Waugh RC, Chanfour X, Yu W. Type III and IV endoleak toward a complete definition of blood flow in the sac after endoluminal AAA repair. J Endovasc Surg 1998; 5:305–309.

7. Riepe G, Heilberger P, Unscheid T, Chakfe N, Raithel D, Stelter W, et al. Frame dislocation of body middle rings in endovascular stent tube grafts. Eur J Vasc Endovasc Surg 1999; 17:28–34.

8. Bohm T, Soldner J, Rott A, Kaiser WA. Perigraft leak of an aortic stent graft due to material fatigue. AJR Am J Roentgenol 1999; 172:1355–1357.

9. Krohg-Sorensen K, Brekke M, Drolsum A, Kvernebo K. Periprosthetic leak and rupture after endovascular repair of abdominal aortic aneurysm; the significance of device design for long-term results. J Vasc Surg 1999; 29:1152–1158.

10. May J. Symposium on distortion and structural deterioration of endovascular grafts used to repair abdominal aortic aneurysms. J Endovasc Surg 1999; 6:1–3.

11. Resch T, Ivancev K, Lindh M, Nyman U, Brunkwall J, Malina M, et al. Persistent collateral perfusion of the abdominal aneurysm after endovascular repair does not lead to progressive change in aneurysm diameter. J Vasc Surg 1998; 28:242–249.

12

Management of Endoleaks After Endovascular Aneurysm Repair

S. William Stavropoulos and Ronald M. Fairman
University of Pennsylvania School of Medicine and University of Pennsylvania Medical Center, Philadelphia, Pennsylvania, U.S.A.

Richard A. Baum
Brigham & Women's Hospital and Harvard Medical School, Boston, Massachusetts, U.S.A.

Endoluminal placement of stent grafts to treat abdominal aortic aneurysms (AAA) shows promising initial results (18,19,36,38,39,42–44). However, the long-term effectiveness of stent grafts is not well known. Endoleaks, which do not occur after traditional aneurysm repair, are detected in approximately 24% of patients undergoing endovascular treatment of AAAs (3–12,15–17,31,32,41). Endoleaks can be difficult to detect and treat, and their management provides new challenges for physicians treating AAAs using an endovascular approach.

I. CLASSIFICATION

The initial endoleak classification system described by White et al., has evolved to include four categories based on their point of origin (47). A leak at an attachment site of the stent graft with the native arterial wall is classified as Type I. This type of endoleak is uncommon, occurring in 3–5% of patients. Type I leaks allow for direct communication between the aneurysm sac and the systemic arterial circulation.

In collateral endoleaks (Type II), blood travels from a branch vessel off of the nonstented portion of the aorta or iliac arteries. Blood flows in a circuitous route, emptying into the aneurysm sac via retrograde flow usually through a lumbar artery or through the inferior mesenteric artery (IMA). This is the most common type of leak and occurs in 20% of patients. Type II leaks are unrelated to the type or configuration of the stent graft.

Endoleaks due to a mechanical problem with the stent graft are referred to as Type III leaks. Fractures, holes, and separation of graft components fall into this category. Today, Type III leaks are rare, but as stent grafts age and long-term follow up is accrued, it is likely that we will see more of these leaks in the future.

Type IV endoleaks are due to stent graft wall porosity. These leaks are identified at the time of implantation when patients are fully anticoagulated. No treatment is needed other than normalizing the patient's coagulation profile.

II. DIAGNOSIS

Evaluation for the presence of endoleaks begins as soon as the stent graft is placed and continues throughout the patient's life. Immediately after deployment of the stent graft an angiogram is performed to evaluate for stent graft placement and the development of an endoleak. If found on the initial post deployment angiogram, Type I and Type III endoleaks are treated immediately in the endovascular suite. Type IV endoleaks are dealt with by reversing the effects of the heparin, which is given during the procedure. Type II endoleaks are followed with a 30-day postoperative computed tomography (CT) scan if seen on the initial postdeployment angiogram.

CT is a sensitive method for evaluating for delayed endoleaks. Duplex ultrasound has also been used (1,2,13,14,21,22,25,26,34,46). At our institution, surveillance CT is used to identify endoleaks. A CT scan is performed 30 days after stent graft deployment on all patients. If this 30-day CT is negative, follow-up CT scans are performed 6 months after stent graft placement and then every 12 months for the duration of the patient's life.

Utilizing proper CT technique is critically important when attempting to detect an endoleak. Noncontrast CT images are first obtain on all patients. These images help to identify areas of calcification, which can have a similar appearance to a small endoleak on contrast enhanced CT. CT angiograms are then performed following the administration of 150 cc of Omnipaque 300 nonionic iodinated contrast agent at 4 cc/s using spiral 3 mm cuts with a pitch of 2. The dynamic CT angiogram images obtained initially can miss some small endoleaks. Therefore, delayed CT images are obtained 5 minutes after initial contrast administration.

If an endoleak is detected on any of the follow-up CT scans, conventional contrast angiography is performed to determine the cause (10). Digital subtraction angiography is performed with a 5 Fr pigtail catheter placed at the proximal attachment site. Anterior-posterior and lateral views are obtained. Filming is performed at 3 frames per second, and filming is continued until contrast has washed out of the arterial and venous system. Similar angiograms are performed with the catheter placed at the graft-to-graft attachment sites. Once anchoring site and graft-to-graft endoleaks are excluded, selective superior mesenteric artery (SMA) and internal iliac artery angiograms are obtained looking for Type II endoleaks. These selective injections are often needed to identify the collateral pathways back to the aneurysm sac via the IMA and lumbar arteries.

Approximately 3–5% of patients will be unable to undergo post-operative CT angiograms because of renal failure as defined by serum creatinine levels greater that 2.5. These patients can be followed with magnetic resonance angiography (MRA) instead of CT (23,28–30,45). Once an endoleak has been detected using MRA, angiography to diagnose which type of endoleak is present can be performed using carbon dioxide or Gadolinium as the arterial contrast agent.

III. TREATMENT

The method of treating endoleaks is determined by the cause of the endoleak, as demonstrated on the angiogram. Attachment site endoleaks (Type I) are repaired immediately after diagnosis. These leaks can be corrected by securing the attachment sites with angioplasty balloons, stents, or stent graft extensions.

The treatment of Type II endoleaks is a source of continuing discussion and debate (9,20,24,27,33,35,37,40). Some consider Type II endoleaks to be insignificant and believe that they should be simply followed indefinitely as long as the aneurysm does not increase in size. The proponents of this view believe that the small collateral vessels that are responsible for Type II leaks are not capable of transmitting arterial pressure to the aneurysm sac. They believe that these small vessels will thrombose spontaneously and only need to be fixed if the aneurysm sac increases in size. Others feel that Type II leaks should be repaired because these small collateral vessels are able to transmit arterial pressure to the aneurysm sac and place the patient at risk for aneurysm rupture. This view is supported by research that demonstrated systemic arterial pressure in the aneurysm sac of patients with Type II endoleaks. At our institution, if a Type II endoleak is seen at 30 days, it is followed until the 6-month CT scan. If it is not seen on the 6-month CT scan, the patient is followed according to our standard protocol. If the leak persists on the 6-month CT scan, the patient is referred for endoleak repair.

The treatment of Type II endoleaks can be performed through a transarterial approach or direct endoleak puncture (9). Using the transarterial technique, a catheter is placed in the vessel of origin, usually the SMA or internal iliac artery. Microcatheters are then manipulated through the collateral vessels into the vessel that communicates with the aneurysm sac, usually the IMA or a lumbar artery. Metallic coils are then used to embolize the vessel near its communication with the aneurysm sac to block the retrograde flow of blood. This procedure can be difficult and time-consuming and is not possible in all patients because of anatomical limitations. In addition, the long-term success of this procedure in embolizing Type II endoleaks has recently come into question. Baum et al. showed that 16 of 20 (80%) Type II endoleaks treated in a transarterial fashion recurred (9). This is because endoleaks are complex vascular structures with multiple feeding and draining vessels, similar to a vascular malformation. Using a transarterial approach, only one branch of the endoleak is embolized. The ingress of the leak is able to shift to a lumbar branch and recanilize the endoleak.

A second and more durable technique for Type II endoleak embolization can be performed using a translumbar approach. With a mean follow-up of 1 year, Baum et al. reported no recurrent Type II endoleaks in 12 translumbar embolizations (9). This technique involves placing patients in the prone position under conscious sedation and with local anesthesia. Prophylactic antibiotics are given intravenously immediately prior to the start of the procedure. Endoleaks identified on prior CT angiography are referenced to bony landmarks and stent graft marking bars. Fluoroscopy of the stent graft is then performed in multiple projections for orientation purposes. Once the access site is identified it can be prepped and draped in the standard fashion. A 19-gauge 20 cm needle with a 5 French (F) Teflon sheath is then inserted through the flank region at the level of the aortic leak and approximately 4 to 5 fingers' breadth from midline. The sheathed needle is advanced under fluoroscopic guidance at a 45–60 degree angle in the antero-medial direction so as to pass just anterior to a vertebral body and just above or below a transverse process. The proper positioning of the catheter within the endoleak is usually signaled by free and pulsatile return of blood and opacification of lumbar arteries or the IMA on manual injection of 5–10 mL of contrast. Once position in the endoleak is confirmed, the translumbar catheter can be used to take pressure measurements and to embolize the endoleak. Embolization can then be performed with coils or "glue." Embolization should continue until there is no further blood return and a static column of contrast is seen on follow-up angiogram of the aneurysm sac.

Endoleaks due to a defect in or failure of the graft material (Type III) provide direct communication between systemic arterial blood and the aneurysm sac and are therefore fixed immediately upon diagnosis. Type III endoleaks can usually be corrected by covering the defect with a stent graft extension.

Type IV endoleaks are uncommon but are usually seen during the immediate postdeployment angiogram while the patients are fully anti-coagulated with heparin. These leaks are self-limited, and treatment consists of normalizing the patient's coagulation status with protamine.

IV. CONCLUSION

Despite recent advances, the management and treatment of endoleaks remains a work in progress. There is general agreement on the need to expeditiously treat patients with Type I and Type III endoleaks. No such consensus exists for the management of Type II endoleaks. Although some Type II leaks have been demonstrated to spontaneously thrombose, the reports of continued AAA enlargement from untreated Type II endoleaks are accumulating. The need to aggressively treat Type II leaks is supported by the recent study measuring pressures within the aneurysm sacs of patients with Type II leaks. This study revealed that systemic arterial pressures in the aneurysm sac were found in all patients with patent Type II endoleaks. This was a dramatic finding, which drives our institutional philosophy of aggressively treating Type II endoleaks. At this time there remains a number of unanswered questions regarding the management of endoleaks. Continued research will help further define when and how patients with endoleaks are managed following stent graft placement.

REFERENCES

1. Abbott WM. Symposium on transluminally placed endovascular prostheses, Bethesda, Maryland, USA, 24–26 March 1994. Introduction and overview. Cardiovasc Surg 1995; 3(2):97–99.

2. Ahn SS, Rutherford RB, Johnston KW, May J, Veith FJ, Baker JD, Ernst CB, Moore WS. Reporting standards for infrarenal endovascular abdominal aortic aneurysm repair. Ad Hoc Committee for Standardized Reporting Practices in Vascular Surgery of The Society for Vascular Surgery/International Society for Cardiovascular Surgery. J Vasc Surg 1997; 25(2):405–410.

3. Aquino RV, Rhee RY, Muluk SC, Tzeng EY, Carrol NM, Makaroun MS. Exclusion of accessory renal arteries during endovascular repair of abdominal aortic aneurysms. J Vasc Surg 2001; 34(5):878–884.

4. Arko FR, Rubin GD, Johnson BL, Hill BB, Fogarty TJ, Zarins CK. Type-II endoleaks following endovascular AAA repair: preoperative predictors and long-term effects. J Endovasc ther 2001; 8(5):503–510.

5. Armon MP, Yusuf SW, Whitaker SC, Gregson RH, Wenham PW, Hopkinson BR. Thrombus distribution and changes in aneurysm size following endovascular aortic aneurysm repair. Eur J Vasc Endovasc Surg 1998; 16(6):472–476.

6. Bade MA, Ohki T, Cynamon J, Veith FJ. Hypogastric artery aneurysm rupture after endovascular graft exclusion with shrinkage of the aneurysm: significance of endotension from a "virtual," or thrombosed type II endoleak. J Vasc Surg 2001; 33(6):1271–1274.

7. Balm R, Jacobs MJ. Use of spiral computed tomographic angiography in monitoring abdominal aortic aneurysms after transfemoral endovascular repair. Texas Heart Inst J 1997; 24(3):200–203.

8. Baum RA, Carpenter JP, Cope C, Golden MA, Velazquez OC, Neschis DG, Mitchell ME, Barker CF, Fairman RM. Aneurysm sac pressure measurements after endovascular repair of abdominal aortic aneurysms. J Vasc Surg 2001; 33(1):32–41.

9. Baum RA, Carpenter JP, Golden MA, Velazquez OC, Clark TW, Stavropoulos SW, Cope C, Fairman RM. Treatment of type 2 endoleaks after endovascular repair of abdominal aortic aneurysms: comparison of transarterial and translumbar techniques. J Vasc Surg 2002; 35(1):23–29.

10. Baum RA, Carpenter JP, Stavropoulos SW, Fairman RM. Diagnosis and management of type 2 endoleaks after endovascular aneurysm repair. Tech Vasc Interv Radiol 2001; 4(4):222–226.

11. Baum RA, Carpenter JP, Tuite CM, Velazquez OC, Soulen MC, Barker CF, Golden MA, Pyeron AM, Fairman RM. Diagnosis and treatment of inferior mesenteric arterial endoleaks after endovascular repair of abdominal aortic aneurysms. Radiology 2000; 215(2):409–413.

12. Baum RA, Cope C, Fairman RM, Carpenter JP. Translumbar embolization of type 2 endoleaks after endovascular repair of abdominal aortic aneurysms. J Vasc Interv Radiol 2001; 12(1):111–116.

13. Beebe HG, Bernhard VM, Parodi JC, White GH. Leaks after endovascular therapy for aneurysm: detection and classification. J Endovasc Surg 1996; 3(4):445–448.

14. Beebe HG, Bernhard VM, Parodi JC, White GH. Leaks after endovascular therapy for aneurysm: detection and classification [see comments]. J Endovasc Surg 1996; 3(4):445–448.
15. Brewster DC, Geller SC, Kaufman JA, Cambria RP, Gertler JP, LaMuraglia GM, Atamian S, Abbott WM. Initial experience with endovascular aneurysm repair: comparison of early results with outcome of conventional open repair. J Vasc Surg 1998; 27(6):992–1005.
16. Chan CL, Ray SA, Taylor PR, Fraser SC, Giddings AE. Endoleaks following conventional open abdominal aortic aneurysm repair. Eur J Vasc Endovasc Surg 2000; 19(3):313–317.
17. Chavan A, Cohnert TU, Heine J, Dresler C, Leuwer M, Harringer W, Jorgensen M, Haverich A, Galanski M. Endoluminal grafting of abdominal aortic aneurysms: experience with the Talent endoluminal stent graft. Eur Radiol 2000; 10(4):636–641.
18. Chuter TA, Donayre C, Wendt G. Bifurcated stent-grafts for endovascular repair of abdominal aortic aneurysm. Preliminary case reports. Surg Endosc 1994; 8(7):800–802.
19. Chuter TA, Green RM, Ouriel K, Fiore WM, DeWeese JA. Transfemoral endovascular aortic graft placement [see comments]. J Vasc Surg 1993; 18(2):185–197.
20. Curti T, Stella A, Rossi C, Galaverni C, Sacca A, Resta F, D'Addato M. Endovascular repair as first-choice treatment for anastomotic and true iliac aneurysms. J Endovasc Ther 2001; 8(2):139–143.
21. Dorffner R, Thurnher S, Prokesch R, Youssefzadeh S, Holzenbein T, Lammer J. Spiral CT during selective accessory renal artery angiography: assessment of vascular territory before aortic stent-grafting. Cardiovasc Intervent Radiol 1998; 21(2):179–182.
22. Dorffner R, Thurnher S, Youssefzadeh S, Winkelbauer F, Holzenbein T, Polterauer P, Lammer J. Spiral CT angiography in the assessment of abdominal aortic aneurysms after stent grafting: value of maximum intensity projections. J Comput Assist Tomogr 1997; 21(3):472–477.
23. Engellau L, Larsson EM, Albrechtsson U, Jonung T, Ribbe E, Thorne J, Zdanowski Z, Norgren L. Magnetic resonance imaging and MR angiography of endoluminally treated abdominal aortic aneurysms. Eur J Vasc Endovasc Surg 1998; 15(3):212–219.
24. Gilling-Smith GL, Martin J, Sudhindran S, Gould DA, McWilliams RG, Bakran A, Brennan JA, Harris PL. Freedom from endoleak after endovascular aneurysm repair does not equal treatment success. Eur J Vasc Endovasc Surg 2000; 19(4):421–425.
25. Golzarian J, Dussaussois L, Abada HT, Gevenois PA, Van Gansbeke D, Ferreira J, Struyven J. Helical CT of aorta after endoluminal stent-graft therapy: value of biphasic acquisition. Am J Roentgenol 1998; 171(2):329–331.

26. Golzarian J, Dussaussois L, Abada HT, Gevenois PA, Van Gansbeke D, Ferreira J, Struyven J. Helical CT of aorta after endoluminal stent-graft therapy: value of biphasic acquisition [see comments]. Am J Roentgenol 1998; 171(2):329–331.

27. Haulon S, Willoteaux S, Kousssa M, Gaxotte V, Beregi JP, Warembourg H. Diagnosis and treatment of type II endoleak after stent placement for exclusion of an abdominal aortic aneurysm. Ann Vasc Surg 2001; 15(2):148–154.

28. Hilfiker PR, Pfammatter T, Lachat M. Depiction of an endoleak after abdominal aortic stent-grafting with contrast-enhanced three-dimensional MR angiography. Am J Roentgenol 1999; 172(2):558.

29. Hilfiker PR, Quick HH, Pfammatter T, Schmidt M, Debatin JF. Three-dimensional MR angiography of a nitinol-based abdominal aortic stent graft: assessment of heating and imaging characteristics. Eur Radiol 1999; 9(9):1775–1780.

30. Hilfiker PR, Quick HH, Schmidt M, Debatin JF. In vitro image characteristics of an abdominal aortic stent graft: CTA versus 3D MRA. Magma 1999; 8(1):27–32.

31. Howell MH, Strickman N, Mortazavi A, Hallman CH, Krajcer Z. Preliminary results of endovascular abdominal aortic aneurysm exclusion with the AneuRx stent-graft. J Am Coll Cardiol 2001; 38(4):1040–1046.

32. Jacobowitz GR, Rosen RJ, Riles TS. The significance and management of the leaking endograft. Semin Vasc Surg 1999; 12(3):199–206.

33. Karch LA, Henretta JP, Hodgson KJ, Mattos MA, Ramsey DE, McLafferty RB, Sumner DS. Algorithm for the diagnosis and treatment of endoleaks. Am J Surg 1999; 178(3):225–231.

34. Krysl J, Vesely TM. Stent graft for treatment of an abdominal aortic aneurysm: leak detected by CT. Am J Roentgenol 1995; 165(3):659–661.

35. Liewald F, Ermis C, Gorich J, Halter G, Scharrer-Pamler R, Sunder-Plassmann L. Influence of treatment of type II leaks on the aneurysm surface area. Eur J Vasc Endovasc Surg 2001; 21(4):339–343.

36. Marin ML, Veith FJ. Images in clinical medicine. Transfemoral repair of abdominal aortic aneurysm. N Engl J Med 1994; 331(26):1751.

37. Martin ML, Dolmatch BL, Fry PD, Machan LS. Treatment of type II endoleaks with Onyx. J Vasc Interv Radiol 2001; 12(5):629–632.

38. May J, White G, Waugh R, Yu W, Harris J. Treatment of complex abdominal aortic aneurysms by a combination of endoluminal and extraluminal aortofemoral grafts. J Vasc Surg 1994; 19(5):924–933.

39. May J, White GH, Waugh RC, Yu W, Stephen MS, Harris JP. Endoluminal repair of abdominal aortic aneurysms. Med J Aust 1994; 161(9):541–543.

40. Mehta M, Ohki T, Veith FJ, Lipsitz EC. All sealed endoleaks are not the same: a treatment strategy based on an ex-vivo analysis. Eur J Vasc Endovasc Surg 2001; 21(6):541–544.

41. Parent FN, Meier GH, Godziachvili V, Lesar CJ, Parker FM, Carter KA, Gayle RG, Demasi RJ, Marcinczyk MJ, Gregory RT. The incidence and natural history of type I and II endoleak: a 5-year follow-up assessment with color duplex ultrasound scan. J Vasc Surg 2002; 35(3):474–481.

42. Parodi JC, Criado FJ, Barone HD, Schonholz C, Queral LA. Endoluminal aortic aneurysm repair using a balloon-expandable stent-graft device: a progress report. Ann Vasc Surg 1994; 8(6):523–529.

43. Parodi JC, Palmaz JC, Barone HD. Transfemoral intraluminal graft implantation for abdominal aortic aneurysms. Ann Vasc Surg 1991; 5(6):491–499.

44. Sayers RD, Thompson MM, Bell PR. Endovascular stenting of abdominal aortic aneurysms. Eur J Vasc Surg 1993; 7(3):225–227.

45. Thurnher SA, Dorffner R, Thurnher MM, Winkelbauer FW, Kretschmer G, Polterauer P, Lammer J. Evaluation of abdominal aortic aneurysm for stent-graft placement: comparison of gadolinium-enhanced MR angiography versus helical CT angiography and digital subtraction angiography. Radiology 1997; 205(2):341–352.

46. Tillich M, Hausegger KA, Tiesenhausen K, Tauss J, Groell R, Szolar DH. Helical CT angiography of stent-grafts in abdominal aortic aneurysms: morphologic changes and complications. Radiographics 1999; 19(6):1573–1583.

47. White GH, May J, Waugh RC, Yu W. Type I and Type II endoleaks: a more useful classification for reporting results of endoluminal AAA repair [letter] [see comments]. J Endovasc Surg 1998; 5(2):189–191.

13
Opinions on Endoleaks

Timothy A. M. Chuter
University of California at San Francisco, San Francisco, California, U.S.A.

I. INTRODUCTION

It is assumed that endovascular repair changes the natural history of aortic aneurysm by excluding the aneurysm from the circulation and protecting its walls from pressure, thereby preventing dilatation and rupture. Freedom from continued aneurysm perfusion is therefore regarded as an indicator of successful endovascular aneurysm repair. The occasional case of aneurysm rupture in the absence of endoleak (1–3) shakes these assumptions and deprives us of a reliable surrogate goal. This consensus conference is part of the academic response to the resulting discomfort. However, the subject is broader than the title would suggest. Our subject is not endoleak, but the efficacy of endovascular aneurysm repair, and we are unlikely to achieve real consensus until we understand the behavior of a new form of arterial pathology, *the graft-lined aortic aneurysm.*

II. ENDOLEAK AS A PREDICTOR OF ANEURYSM RUPTURE

Elective aneurysm repair is a prophylactic operation, intended to prevent death from aneurysm rupture. Endovascular aneurysm repair is a success when the patient dies of an unrelated disease, and a failure when the patient dies of aneurysm rupture or of complications following endovascular

135

treatment. Alternative measures of success are of no value as surrogate goals unless they reliably predict one of these definitive outcomes.

There have been many reported instances of aneurysm rupture in the absence of endoleak (1–3). These lapses in the predictive value of endoleak have prompted a reevaluation of the effects of a stent-graft, a search for other more predictive findings, and the adoption of new concepts, such as endotension (4). Some authors have even gone so far as to suggest that the occurrence of endoleak bears no relation to the incidence of aneurysm rupture (1). In my opinion, this is premature.

Any patient with a ruptured aneurysm certainly has an endoleak, and in most cases this endoleak was apparent on earlier imaging. Based on Eurostar data (5), an endoleak of type I or III is associated with a greater than 10-fold increase in the risk of rupture. However, aneurysms do occasionally rupture in the absence of a known endoleak. This occurrence may be explained in a variety of ways.

1. The diagnosis of endoleak is entirely image-based, and the accuracy depends on the imaging technique. Type II endoleaks are easily missed unless data acquisition includes a delayed phase, and are easily confused with distal aortic calcification unless there is a noncontrast series for comparison.
2. The position of the device may be unstable, resulting in a sudden transition from sealed and protective to leaking and nonprotective. For example, bowing or kinking of the limbs can lead to dislocation of the iliac end into the aneurysm or dislocation of the stent-graft junction, resulting in a large endoleak. Hence the relationship between kinking and risk of rupture. This is a characteristic failure mode of devices, such as Vanguard, with long flexible limbs (6). Alternatively, the proximal end of the stent-graft sometimes flips out of a short angulated neck, with similar results (3). This is a characteristic failure mode of rigid devices, such as the AneuRx, that lack barbs or suprarenal fixation.
3. The structural integrity of the device may be unstable, resulting in type III leakage, which is sometimes sudden and catastrophic, and sometimes subacute and intermittent. The prime example of the structurally unstable stent-graft was the Vanguard (6), which was prone to disruption of the Nitinol endoskeleton, leading to fabric erosion and rupture. More subtle problems affect porous devices such as AneuRx (7). According to core lab data, 50% of cases showed signs of endoleak at the time of discharge. This number fell to 15% at

one month. Most of the early leaks were categorized as a type IV (9), which were regarded as more benign than other forms of transgraft leakage (type III endoleak). However, the thrombus that seals many type IV leaks may not be as durable, or as protective, as was once supposed. Certainly, thrombosis of a type 1 endoleak offers no protection. These leaks recur and the aneurysms rupture. I suspect that something of the sort may occur with type IV endoleaks. First, patients treated with less porous devices, such as Ancure (8), show more aneurysm shrinkage than patients treated with more porous devices, such as AneuRx (7). Second, the AneuRx device sometimes appears at the time of conversion, to resemble a fountain with one or more little holes spraying blood into the aneurysm. It is unclear whether these findings result from the initial porosity of the device or from the long-term effects of repetitive strain.

III. ENDOLEAK AND ANEURYSM DILATATION

Patients who show signs of continued pressurization of the aneurysm sac are said to have "endotension." The term is often applied to patients who have enlarging aneurysms with (4) or without endoleak (10). The existence of elevated pressure in these cases is entirely hypothetical since there is rarely any means of actually measuring pressure. In many cases unexplained aneurysm dilatation (endotension) probably represents the residual effect of a sealed endoleak, in which a short, wide plug of thrombus is the only barrier between the arterial lumen and the aneurysm sac. This phenomenon was more common in the days when aorto-aortic stent-grafts were sometimes implanted distally in a cuff of thrombus rather than nondilated aorta. Another recently described cause of endotension is low-grade infection of the aneurysm contents.

Personally, I avoid the term *endotension* because it tells us very little about etiology, prognosis, or treatment. Moreover, it implies a cause, aneurysm pressurization, for which there is no evidence, except in cases of endoleak (11,12).

We know as little about the process by which some aneurysms shrink as we do about the causes of aneurysm dilatation. It is comforting to see a decline in aneurysm diameter, but this probably does not represent any kind of healing. Years after a successful endovascular aneurysm repair and a steady decline in aneurysm diameter, the development of a delayed endoleak will be associated with an almost instantaneous return to the original size. Indeed, Parodi has suggested that successful endovascular repair may cause the wall of the aneurysm to atrophy, placing the patient at even greater risk of rupture when the endovascular barrier fails. Nevertheless, aneurysms generally shrink when an endoleak is absent from the outset (8) or is treated (13), indicating that the expected link between aneurysm perfusion and aneurysm dilatation does exist.

Aneurysm volume has been suggested as a more sensitive measure of changing aneurysm size than aneurysm diameter (14), but the difference hardly justifies the additional effort while so little is known about the causes and significance of aneurysm dilatation or shrinkage.

IV. ENDOLEAK AND THE ANEURYSM PULSE

An untreated aneurysm is a large, compliant reservoir. While the aneurysm lumen remains connected to the central arterial circulation, its wall moves back and forth through a wide excursion in response to the pressure changes of the arterial waveform. The resulting pulsation only occurs if large quantities of blood are free to move in and out of the aneurysm sac, and pulsation is diminished when the stent-graft provides an effective barrier to flow between the circulation and the aneurysm. Therefore, the aneurysm pulse, as assessed by gated ultrasound measurements (15), remains prominent when blood sloshes to-and-fro through a large type I or type III endoleak and may disappear altogether when there is no endoleak. As one might expect, type II endoleaks occupy an intermediate position. These endoleaks also sustain the pulse by providing a route in and out of the aneurysm, but this effect is probably modest because so little blood can flow through the typical type II pathway in the short time between systole and diastole. A more important effect is the ability of a type II endoleak to maintain the volume (and pressure) of the perigraft space. If the pressure in this space exceeds arterial pressure at any point in the cardiac cycle the wall of the stent-graft will flap, and it is the flapping of a compliant stent-graft that produces most of the volume changes felt as aneurysm pulsation. This type of flapping of the stent-graft wall is commonly seen on intraoperative fluoroscopy. As a result, it is rare for there to be a striking change in aneurysm pulse immediately after endovascular aneurysm repair, despite the observed fall in aneurysm pressure (12).

V. THE DIAGNOSIS OF ENDOLEAK

In my opinion, a contrast-enhanced spiral computed tomography (CT), with both an arterial phase and a delayed data acquisition, is very sensitive for endoleak. The specificity is enhanced by an initial noncontrast study. Although anatomical detail is sometimes lacking, I believe these studies are usually sufficient to differentiate type I from type II endoleak. Most type II endoleaks are distal and easily distinguished from proximal type I endoleaks. Distal type I endoleaks are more difficult to diagnose on CT images alone, especially if the area is heavily calcified. However, this type of endoleak is quite rare if one uses a system with a large range of distal stent-graft diameters and configurations.

The distinction between type II endoleaks and those of types I and III is very important, because each has a different prognosis. Type II endoleaks are benign while the others lead to rupture. If any doubt exists, an angiogram will usually settle the issue. Type I endoleaks fill promptly from one end of the aneurysm or the other, whereas type III endoleaks fill shortly after infusion of contrast into the central portion of the stent-graft. Type II endoleaks fill much later and may require selective injection for proper visualization. Angiography is not necessarily a reliable indicator of the direction of flow within a collateral pathway because the infusion of contrast promotes flow from the tip of the catheter into the aneurysm. Moreover, the direction of flow through collateral routes sometimes varies according to the patient's position.

VI. PREVENTION AND TREATMENT OF ENDOLEAK

Most instances of proximal type I endoleak result from errors in patient selection. The neck is too short, too angulated, or too irregular for proper stent-graft implantation. A type I endoleak is very rare in patients who meet the stated selection criteria for the device. Unfortunately, the patients who most need endovascular aneurysm repair often lack the desired anatomy and one is forced to risk type I leakage. Sometimes it is possible to treat the leak by forcing the neck into more favorable configuration using a giant Palmaz stent. Alternatively, the neck can be cinched down on the stent-graft using an external ligature. I do not believe that anything is to be gained by filling a type I endoleak with coils. The endoleak may disappear, but the risk of rupture will persist. Stent-graft extension in the proximal direction is usually limited by the proximity of the renal arteries, although this limitation may eventually be surmounted by the development of fenestrated and multibranched stent-grafts (16,17).

Distal type I endoleak is usually treatable by extending the conduit into the external iliac artery. This option carries greater risks when both common iliac arteries are unsuitable for stent-graft implantation.

Type II endoleaks are difficult to predict, prevent, and treat, but fortunately most appear relatively benign (18). Most patients have patent lumbar arteries on preoperative studies, many show signs of type II endoleak on intraoperative angiograms, and many of these (approximately 20%) will have type II endoleak on postoperative CT, yet very few experience aneurysm dilatation or rupture. Indeed, the Eurostar data show no correlation between the presence of type II endoleak and the risk of rupture (5).

The strongest predictors of type II endoleak are preoperative coumadin therapy and a paucity of mural thrombus. However, the risk of type II endoleak hardly justifies excluding a patient from endovascular aneurysm repair.

Intraoperative aneurysm packing with thrombin-soaked gelatin sponges seems to be effective but is too time-consuming for routine use. Polymer infusion holds promise as a quicker, easier way to achieve the same effect.

There are three possible routes to the site of leakage: through the feeding arteries from the SMA or internal iliac artery; between the orifice of the stent-graft and the surrounding artery; and directly into the aneurysm by translumbar puncture. The first of these is the most widely used. It is often possible to pass a catheter through the superior mesenteric artery (SMA), around the colonic arterial arcade, and through the inferior mesenteric artery (IMA) all the way to the aneurysm for coil embolization (19). One might expect that embolization of the feeding artery would be definitive treatment for type II leakage. Although there are often many routes into the aneurysm through lumbar arteries, these are more difficult to catheterize. The ascending branches of the internal iliac artery often feed the lumbar arteries through a network of tiny vessels. Coiling all these vessels not only fails to eliminate the leak, it also risks compromising the arterial supply of the lumbosacral plexus. Aggressive internal iliac/lumbar embolization can cause paralysis.

The group at the University of Pennsylvania were the fist to describe translumbar endoleak embolization. This approach appears to be effective in the short-to-medium term.

We used to treat all endoleaks within a month or two after stent-graft implantation (18). Our attempts to treat type II endoleaks were largely ineffective; the branched vessels were successfully embolized, but the leaks persisted. Yet only two patients showed signs of aneurysm dilatation. Both had leakage through IMA collaterals (18). Consequently, we now treat IMA and lumbar leaks differently. The IMA endoleaks are treated promptly, but the lumbar leaks are observed. In the past 2 years, since adopting this policy, we have seen nothing to make us doubt the safety of this approach. It is sometimes difficult to make the distinction between lumbar and IMA endoleaks on CT alone, but in most cases the IMA-related endoleaks are anterior and proximal, while the lumbar artery-related leaks are posterior and distal.

Primary type III endoleaks usually result from faulty implantation technique. These are rare and easily corrected. Secondary type III endoleaks result from faulty stent-graft design. Causative factors include inadequately electro-polished (gray to black) Nitinol stents, flimsy loosely woven fabrics, and isolated load-bearing sutures.

VII. CONCLUSION

There are several reasons why aneurysms rupture in the absence of known endoleak, none of which apply uniformly to all forms of endovascular aneurysm repair; they are device and technique specific. In my opinion, the absence of endoleak can still be relied upon as an indicator of protection from risk of rupture when a durable nonporous stentgraft has been attached securely to nondilated arteries proximal and distal to the aneurysm.

REFERENCES

1. Zarins CK, White RA, Hodgson KJ, et al. Endoleak as a predictor of outcome after endovascular aneurysm repair: AneuRx multicenter clinical trial. J Vasc Surg 2000; 32:90–107.
2. Gilling-Smith G, Martin J, Sudhindran S, et al. Freedom from endoleak after endovascular aneurysm repair does not equal treatment success. Eur J Vasc Endovasc Surg 2000; 19:421–425.
3. Politz JK, Newman VS, Stewart MT. Late abdominal aortic aneurysm rupture after AneuRx repair: a report of three cases. J Vasc Surg 2000; 31:599–606.
4. Gilling-Smith G, Brennan J, Harris P, et al. Endotension after endovascular aneurysm repair: definition, classification, and strategies for surveillance and intervention. J Endovasc Surg 1999; 6:305–307.
5. Harris P. Rupture after endovascular aneurysm repair: implications for clinical practice. Presented Feb 14, 2001, at the Congress of the International Society for Endovascular Specialists, Scottsdale, AZ.
6. Beebe HG, Cronenwett JL, Katzen BT, Brewster DC, et al. Results of an aortic endograft trial: impact of device failure beyond 12 months. J Vasc Surg 2001; 33:S55–63.
7. Zarins CK, White RA, Moll FL, et al. The AneuRx stent graft: four-year results and worldwide experience 2000. J Vasc Surg 2001; 33:S135–145.
8. Makaroun MS. The Ancure endografting system: an update. J Vasc Surg 2001; 33:S129–134.

9. White GH, May J, Waugh, et al. Type III and type IV endoleak: toward a complete definition of blood flow in the sac after endoluminal AAA repair. J Endovasc Surg 1998; 5:305–309.
10. White GH, May J. How should endotension be defined? History of a concept and evolution of a new term. J Endovasc Ther 2000; 7:435–438.
11. Baum RA, Carpenter JP, Cope C, et al. Aneurysm sac pressure measurements after endovascular repair of abdominal aortic aneurysms. J Vasc Surg 2001; 33:32–41.
12. Chuter TAM, Ivancev K, Malina M, et al. Aneurysm pressure following endovascular exclusion. Eur J Vasc Endovasc Surg 1997; 13:85–87.
13. Ermis C, Kramer S, Tomczak R, et al. Does successful embolization of endoleaks lead to aneurysm sac shrinkage? J Endovasc Ther 2000; 7:441–445.
14. Wever JJ, Blankensteijn JD, Mali WPM, Eikelboom B. Maximal aneurysm diameter follow-up is inadequate after endovascular abdominal aortic aneurysm repair. Eur J Vasc Surg 1999; 18:475–480.
15. Malena M, Lanne T, Ivancev K, et al. Reduced pulsatile wall motion of abdominal aortic aneurysms after endovascular repair. J Vasc Surg 1998; 27:631.
16. Anderson JL, Berce M, Hartley DE. Endoluminal aortic grafting with renal and superior mesenteric artery incorporation by graft fenestration. J Endovasc Ther 2001; 8:3–15.
17. Chuter TAM, Gordon RL, Reilly LM, Goodman JD, Messina LM. An endovascular system for thoracoabdominal aortic aneurysm repair. J Endovasc Ther 2001; 8:25–33.
18. Chuter TAM, Faruqi R, Sawhney R, Reilly LM, Kerlan RK, Canto CJ, Lukaszewicz GC, LaBerge JM, Wilson MW, Gordon RL, Wall SD, Rapp J, Messina LM. Endoleak following endovascular repair of abdominal aortic aneurysm. J Vasc Surg 2001; 34:98–105.
19. Baum RA, Carpenter JP, Tuite CM, et al. Diagnosis and treatment of inferior mesenteric arterial endoleaks after endovascular repair of abdominal aortic aneurysms. Radiology 2000; 215:409–413.

14

Endoleak and Endotension: The Springfield Experience

Maurice M. Solis
Macon Cardio-Vascular Institute, Macon, Georgia, U.S.A.

Kim J. Hodgson
Southern Illinois University School of Medicine, Springfield, Illinois, U.S.A.

I. INTRODUCTION

Endoluminal repair of infrarenal abdominal aortic aneurysms (AAA) has become an accepted treatment option for patients with suitable vascular anatomy. Unfortunately, the goal of excluding the aneurysm sac from blood flow is not always achieved. The presence of blood flow outside the lumen of an endovascular graft but within the aneurysm sac or adjacent vascular segments being treated has been termed endoleak and implies some degree of maintained pressurization of the aneurysm sac (1). While some endoleaks (especially types II and III) represent an unexpected sequella of endografting aortic aneurysms, the mechanism of formation is conceptually simple. Contrarily, the mechanism of another new concept, endotension, remains obscure. Endotension refers to the persistent pressurization of the aneurysm sac in the absence of a detectable endoleak (2). Understanding the role of endoleak and endotension in the success or failure of endoluminal aneurysm repair is one of the major challenges facing endovascular specialists.

II. NATURAL HISTORY AND SIGNIFICANCE OF ENDOLEAKS

For many reasons the natural history of endoleaks has been difficult to elucidate. Endoleaks often resolve spontaneously, but they can also appear spontaneously after periods of seemingly complete aneurysm exclusion. To date, the correlation between the presence of an endoleak and aneurysm enlargement is poor, though follow-up intervals are relatively brief (3). Excluded aneurysm sacs are seen to diminish in size despite the presence of an endoleak, yet sometimes they increase in size without a detectable endoleak being present (4). Long-term follow-up to lend guidance about the most effectual way to approach endoleaks is not yet available, which has resulted in a haphazard array of treatments of unknown efficacy. Clearly, many endoleaks can and are now being treated by successful secondary endovascular procedures, though the need for this and the long-term outcome is unknown.

The Society for Vascular Surgery/International Society for Cardiovascular Surgery Ad Hoc Committee on Reporting Standards for Endovascular AAA Repair include the absence of endoleak in their definitions of technical and clinical success of endoluminal aneurysm repair (5). However, the presence of an endoleak is clearly not associated with progressive aneurysm enlargement in most cases (6). The recently published midterm results of the two largest endograft series are illustrative of the current controversy. The latest results from the EUROSTAR (European Collaborators on Stent/Graft Techniques for Aortic Aneurysm Repair) Registry of 2464 patients reported a significantly increased risk of rupture and conversion to open surgical repair for patients with persistent endoleaks (7). In contrast, the latest report of the worldwide experience with the AneuRx endograft system in 1192 patients found that the presence of an endoleak on a follow-up computed tomography (CT) scan was not a predictor of long-term outcome (8,9). Although differences in study design, devices used, and outcomes evaluated can, in some measure, account for the contradictory conclusions, the true significance of endoleak in the long-term results of endograft aneurysm repair remains uncertain.

III. DIAGNOSIS

While CT scanning is currently the gold-standard imaging modality for the detection of postoperative endoleak (Fig. 1), its expense and invasiveness has sparked a demand for a less invasive diagnostic alternative. Much attention

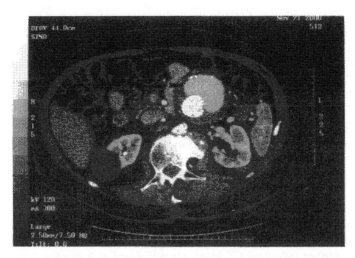

Figure 1. Contrast-enhanced blood flow is easily seen on this CT scan to be outside of the endograft but within the aneurysm sac (arrow), diagnostic of a large endoleak.

has been focused on color duplex ultrasound (CDU) as a possible alternative, though the most appropriate role for color-flow duplex ultrasound in the follow-up evaluation of endograft patients has not been established. While several series have reported excellent correlation with CT scanning (10,11), others have found poor positive predictive values and frequent suboptimal CDU examinations (12). We recently reviewed our experience with CDU in 79 patients who underwent endoluminal AAA repair. CDU correctly detected endoleaks in all six patients with positive CT scans, and there was one false-positive ultrasound examination. As compared to endoleaks detected by CT scanning, CDU had a sensitivity of 100%, specificity of 100%, positive predictive value of 88%, negative predictive value of 100%, and an accuracy of 99% in our series.

Several authors have reported that improved sensitivity with CDU can be achieved by the administration of ultrasonographic contrast agents, frequently detecting endoleaks that had not been noted by contrast-enhanced CT scanning (3,13). Although the results of standard and contrast-enhanced CDU in regards to endoleak detection are promising, we believe that the less accurate diameter measurements and the limited anatomical information obtained by CDU limit its usefulness as the primary imaging modality in the follow-up of endograft repair (14). These parameters are often our only indicators, albeit indirect, of maintained aneurysm pressure. Consequently, while we currently use CDU in the early postoperative period to assess for gross endoleaks indicative of attachment site leakage, we continue to rely upon CT scanning as the primary imaging modality beyond the perioperative period.

The optimal surveillance protocol for patients treated by endoluminal aortic grafting is not known, nor is the length of time that patients will need to be surveyed. The surveillance protocol adopted at Southern Illinois University, and the rationale for it, have been previously reported (15). Currently we recommend that patients undergo CDU prior to discharge to assess for gross problems and either a CDU or CT scan at 1 month. If the imaging at 1 month indicates the presence of an endoleak, a CT scan is performed 3 months postendograft. If an endoleak is still present at 3 months, we evaluate it angiographically to ensure that it is not of the type I or III variety, for which treatment is generally felt to be required. If no endoleak is noted on the 1 month scan, or on the 3-month scan for those positive at 1 month, further follow-up CT scans are performed at 6 months, 1 year, and annually thereafter. More frequent CT scanning may be undertaken in patients who have persistent endoleaks, undergo secondary interventions, or exhibit evidence of aneurysm enlargement.

Indications for angiography at our institution include a primary endoleak still present at 3 months, the development of a secondary endoleak, and persistent aneurysm enlargement with or without an endoleak on CT. An extensive angiographic search for the origin of the endoleak is often required. Flush aortography will usually demonstrate a proximal type I endoleak, while selective angiography of the superior mesenteric artery (SMA) and both internal iliac arteries with prolonged (late-phase) imaging may be needed to delineate a type II endoleak (Fig. 2). Selective contrast injection of the iliac graft limbs and retrograde sheath injections are useful in detecting distal attachment site type I endoleaks. Multiple "directed" contrast injections at the sites of component junctions are sometimes necessary to localize the origin of type III endoleaks (Fig. 3). Some authors have described outflow balloon occlusion of one or both limbs of the endograft to allow a static column of contrast to sit in the graft. This may allow visualization of persistent "microleaks" related to needle-hole bleeding or small fabric defects.

IV. ENDOLEAK MANAGEMENT

The most appropriate method of management of endoleaks remains controversial. The distinct differences in the risks associated with the different types of endoleaks, likely related to the degree of pressurization they impart on the aneurysm sac, render a uniform approach to all endoleaks problematic. Nonetheless, there is a general agreement on the correct approach to many endoleaks and active research into the best approach for others.

A. Type I Endoleaks

A proximal type I endoleak is caused by inadequate sealing of the proximal attachment site of an endovascular graft to the wall of the aneurysm neck. Both the anatomical features of the neck and the technical aspects of endograft implantation are important factors in the development of a proximal endoleak. Proximal type I endoleaks are more common in patients with shorter, larger and severely angulated aneurysm necks, although the presence of thrombus and calcification in the neck does not appear to be as significant a risk factor, as previously thought (16). Self-expanding endografts should be oversized by 10–20%, and balloon "modeling" of the attachment site may assist in obtaining a hemostatic seal, particularly with irregularly contoured necks. Proximal deployment of the graft should be as close to the renal arteries as possible to achieve maximal overlap between the graft and aneurysm neck. Additionally, the use of devices with suprarenal uncovered stent fixation may decrease the incidence of proximal type I endoleak in patients with short (< 10 mm) necks (17). With proper patient and graft selection and accurate graft deployment, the early incidence of proximal type I endoleak is minimized. Still unknown is whether progressive neck dilation following endograft repair will ultimately result in late proximal endoleaks. Aortic neck enlargement in the range of 0.9–1.9 mm per year has been observed in the first 2 years after endovascular grafting (18). Consequently, close long-term patient follow-up remains mandatory in view of the potential risk of late failure as a result of continued expansion of aortic or iliac necks.

Small primary proximal type I endoleaks in a well-positioned graft can be safely followed for the first 3 months and, in our experience, will frequently resolve spontaneously. Patients with persistent primary, or any secondary, proximal type I endoleaks, on the other hand, are at a significant risk of aneurysm enlargement and rupture. In a recent update of the EUROSTAR endograft trial, persistent type I endoleaks were associated with a 4.6% rate of rupture and a combined rupture/conversion rate of 23% (7). Persistent and secondary proximal type I endoleaks are often associated with significant distal migration of the endograft. The development of a late proximal leak should prompt a thorough review of past imaging studies to determine the extent of any graft migration.

All patients with persistent type I endoleaks at the proximal attachment site should be treated to prevent aneurysm rupture. Deployment of a larger diameter proximal endograft extension is the best treatment option in those patients with a sufficient length of uncovered aortic neck between the renal arteries and the cephalad end of the endograft. This approach is ideally suited for, and particularly effective in, those situations where the endograft was deployed low in the neck or has migrated distally. Successful exclusion of the

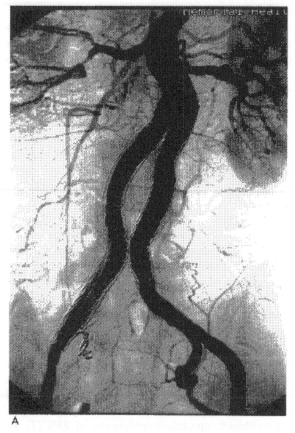

A

Figure 2.   Selective contrast injection of the SMA (B) uncovers a mesenteric type II endoleak (arrowheads) not visualized by flush aortogram (A).

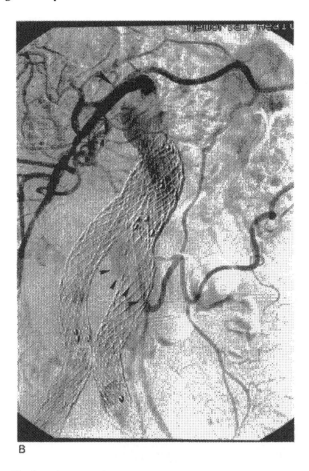

B

Figure 2. Continued.

sac by coil embolization of the proximal perigraft channel has also been
reported in patients without graft migration (19). However, the effectiveness
of this treatment in depressurizing the aneurysm sac is uncertain. Due to the
serious risk of aneurysm rupture in patients with persistent or late type I
endoleaks, serious consideration should also be given to open surgical repair
or at least a more frequent and intensive surveillance protocol.

Distal type I endoleaks are a similar failure of graft to artery attachment,
the usual cause being dilated or calcified common iliac arteries. A few
aneurysm ruptures have been reported in patients with untreated distal type I

endoleaks (20). Although the risk may be less than for proximal endoleaks, treatment of all patients with distal type I endoleaks is clearly indicated (7). Fortunately, most distal type I endoleaks are readily treated by various endovascular techniques, the most common being deployment of distal extension endograft components. Graft extension to the external iliac artery following internal iliac embolization may be required. Alternatively, placing larger-diameter aortic cuffs in a bell-bottom fashion may effectively seal

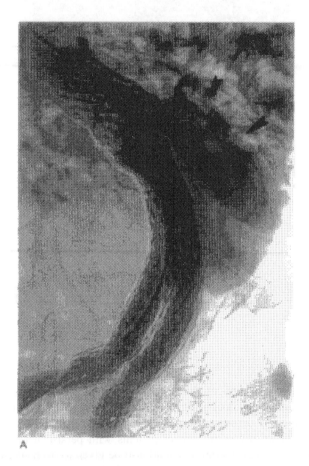

Figure 3. (A) Flush aortogram showing a large endoleak (arrows), the origin of which cannot be clearly ascertained. (B) "Directed" contrast injection demonstrating the exact site of the type III endoleak. Notice the tip of the Simmons-1 catheter protruding between graft components and contrast filling the aneurysm sac (arrows).

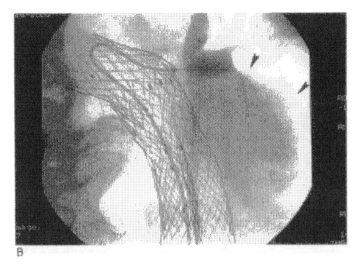

Figure 3. Continued.

enlarged but not aneurysmal common iliac arteries (21). Successful aneurysm exclusion can also be accomplished by coil embolization of the perigraft channel immediately proximal to the distal attachment site (Fig. 4) (16). The effectiveness of this approach likely depends at least somewhat on the length of the channel being embolized, longer embolized tracts being more likely to effectively depressurize the aneurysm sac (22). Recently, banding of the common iliac artery around the endograft limb through a retroperitoneal incision has been described (23).

B. Type II Endoleaks

Angiography performed immediately following endograft implantation commonly demonstrates patent lumbar arteries, opacified either directly through as-yet-unsealed attachment sites or via early graft porosity, or indirectly through mesenteric or ilio-lumbar collaterals. While most of these collateral vessel endoleaks will thrombose in the early postoperative period, continued patency results in a type II endoleak. That any of these collateral blood flow channels persist long term, through the thrombogenic environment of an excluded aneurysm sac partially filled with a large endograft foreign body, is one of the most counterintuitive findings following the endoluminal treatment of aneurysms. Two patterns of collateral blood flow into the

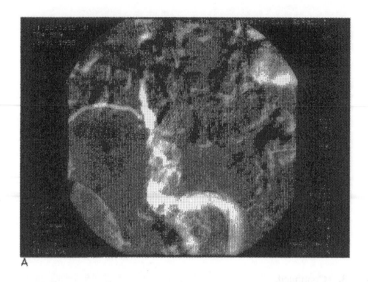

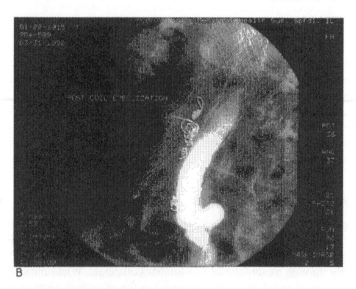

Figure 4. (A) Contrast injection into the perigraft channel of the left iliac landing zone delineating a distal type I endoleak with outflow from a single lumbar artery. (B) Posttreatment angiogram following coil embolization of the outflow lumbar artery and distal perigraft channel. (From Ref. 15.)

aneurysm sac predominate. In the first, blood flows from branches of the internal iliac artery to an ipsilateral lumbar artery (ilio-lumbar type) (Fig. 5). Less commonly, blood flows from the SMA to the inferior mesenteric artery (IMA) via an arc of Riolan or marginal artery (mesenteric type) (Fig. 2). In either case, an outflow vessel, frequently a lumbar artery, must be present to maintain patency of the circuit. The incidence of type II endoleak has been reported to correlate with the preoperative patency of the IMA, as well as the number of patent lumbar arteries (24). Prophylactic embolization is not generally felt to be justified, however, as the preoperative patency of these vessels is not sufficiently predictive of postoperative endoleak (25,26).

The significance of persistent type II endoleaks remains an area of controversy, which is unfortunate because they are the most common type of endoleak encountered. Aneurysm ruptures felt to have been caused by type II endoleaks have been reported (27). In the EUROSTAR series, persistent type II endoleaks were associated with a combined rupture/-conversion rate of 5.3% (7). In animals with surgically constructed type II endoleaks, systemic sac mean and pulse pressures were found to correlate with the diameter of the patent collateral vessel (28). Systemic or near systemic sac pressures have been measured in patients with type II endoleaks by selective SMA to IMA catheterization and by translumbar puncture (29). These hemodynamic investigations strongly support an aggressive approach to obliterating type II endoleaks, though the effectiveness of sac pressure reduction following embolization has not been thoroughly studied.

Since first reported in 1997, coil embolization has emerged as the main treatment of type II endoleak (30). In patients in whom angiography demonstrates a principal collateral vessel from either the SMA or internal iliac artery to the aneurysm sac, microcatheter access to the orifice of the IMA or lumbar artery can be achieved and superselective coil deployment successfully accomplished (Fig. 6) (22,31). While a decrease in aneurysm size after successful embolization has been reported, the efficacy in depressurization of the excluded sac is unproven (32,33). Other techniques for treating type II endoleaks include direct translumbar injection of thrombin into the sac and laparoscopic clipping of the offending collateral vessels (34,35). Prevention of type II endoleaks by the recent innovation of intraoperative packing of the aneurysm sac with collagen sponge appears promising (36). We currently recommend angiography and attempted embolization of all type II endoleaks present at or after 3 months of follow-up. Patients with persistent endoleaks following embolization are retreated at an interval of 6 months, especially if their aneurysm is enlarging.

C. Type III Endoleaks

A type III endoleak represents a mechanical structural failure of an implanted endograft. The most common type III endoleak occurs as a result of loosening and separation of a component-to-component junction in a modular system. Actual fabric defects, another variant of a type III endoleak, have also been reported but appear to occur less commonly (37). Component separation often results from angulation of the endograft at the site of a component junction, often secondary to late conformational changes occurring in the endografted

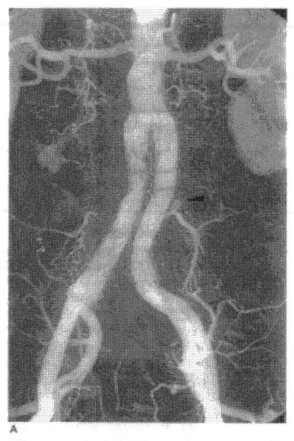

Figure 5. Flush aortogram (A) and selective hypogastric arteriogram (B) demonstrating contrast entering the aneurysm sac (arrows) from ilio-lumbar type II endoleaks.

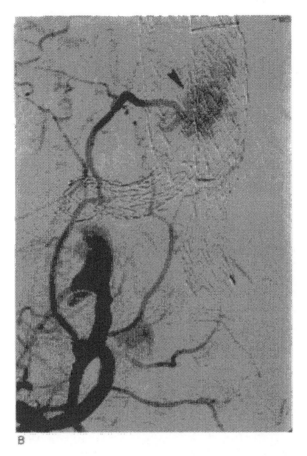

Figure 5. Continued.

aortic aneurysm. Material fatigue and insufficient component overlap may also play a role. Hemodynamically there is usually a sizable direct communication between the endograft lumen and the aneurysm sac, and, as such, endografted aneurysms with type III endoleaks are considered to be pressurized and in need of reintervention. In the EUROSTAR trial, type III endoleaks were associated with a 5.4% risk of rupture and a rupture/conversion risk of almost 20% (7).

Correction of type III endoleaks can often be accomplished by the deployment of another graft component across the area of detachment or fabric defect. Although this can be a straightforward endovascular procedure, the conformational changes that caused the component separation in the first place can complicate the procedure, and custom-made components may be required to achieve successful repair (Fig. 7). In some situations, conversion to the aorto-uni-iliac confirmation with femoral-femoral bypass grafting may be required to exclude the portion of the endograft from which the type II endoleak arises. If a suitable endoluminal repair option is not available, conversion to open surgical repair is mandatory.

D. Type IV Endoleaks

In our experience, type IV or "porosity" endoleak has been an insignificant and self-limiting finding. Faint contrast blushes seen occasionally on

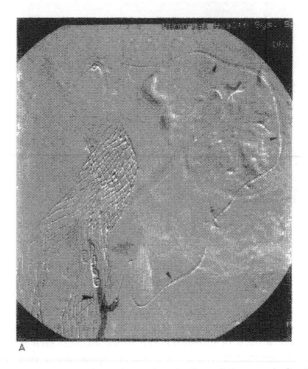

A

Figure 6. (A) Superselective microcatheterization of the marginal artery (small arrowheads) and proximal IMA (large arrowhead) during endoleak coil embolization. (B) Completion SMA angiogram showing obliteration of the mesenteric type II endoleak by microcoils in proximal IMA (arrowhead).

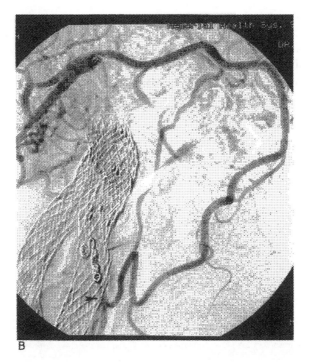

B

Figure 6. Continued.

completion angiogram are presumed to be type IV leaks and invariably resolve, usually prior to discharge. Type IV endoleaks from the puncture site of sutures used to attach the stents to the graft material were observed in an early endograft design subsequently withdrawn from the market (38). Whether the other endograft devices incorporating sutured-on stents will develop these types of endoleaks, either as a result of sutures pulling out, leaving unfilled holes, or due to fabric weave separation from suture traction on the fabric, remains unknown.

E. Endotension

The precise definition of the term endotension is currently a subject of debate (39,40). We find the definition put forward by White et al. the most useful, namely that endotension is the phenomenon of persistent or recurrent pressurization of the aneurysm sac following endoluminal repair without evidence of endoleak (39). Endotension is the presumed cause of continued aneurysm expansion following endoluminal repair despite total exclusion of the sac from the circulation by the endograft. The mechanism by which this unexpected phenomenon occurs is unknown. Endotension has been reported to be the cause of postoperative aneurysm expansion in as many as 18% of patients (3). That aneurysm rupture can occur without a discernable endoleak

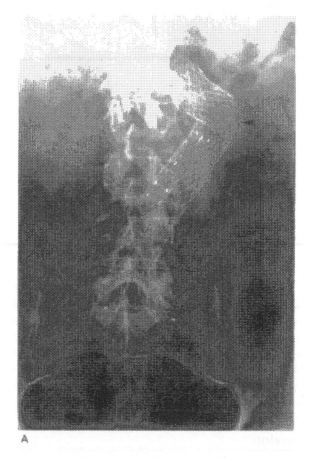

A

Figure 7. (A) Late conformational changes in the neck of an aneurysm resulting in complete separation (arrowhead) of the main endograft body from an aortic extender component. (B) Successful endoluminal repair of the type III endoleak by deployment of a custom-made tube graft component (arrowhead) across the area of separation.

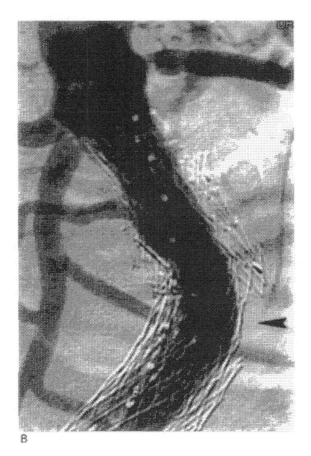

B

Figure 7. Continued.

is unquestionable (3,20), but may simply reflect the fact that an endoleak developed between the time of the last scan and the occurrence of the rupture.

Several possible causes of endotension have been proposed. Transmission of pressure through a small rim or plug of thrombus sealing an endograft attachment site or aortic side branch seems to us the most probable, and some investigational support for this theory can be given (41). Aneurysm expansion without endoleak is often associated with distal migration of the endograft. Furthermore, some endografts explanted secondary to endotension have been found to have poor fixation at one or more attachment sites (20). In vitro and animal studies have indicated that thrombosis of a type I or II endoleak may not significantly decrease the pressure within the excluded sac (20,28). Another likely rationale is that endotension expansion is caused by blood flow into the sac (i.e., endoleak), which is not detectable by current imaging techniques. The sensitivity of CT scanning maybe insufficient to detect very small leaks or leaks in which no outflow vessel is present. Some patients with aneurysm expansion despite no apparent endoleak on CT scan have subsequently had endoleaks detected by contrast-enhanced CDU (3,13). In two patients with elevated intrasac pressures but no endoleak by CT or standard angiography, direct contrast injection into the sac revealed a patent lumbar or IMA (29). Microleaks not detected by CT have also been found during endograft explantation (see below). Finally, though less likely in our opinion, is the possibility that endotension-associated aneurysm expansion is due to biological processes in the diseased aortic segment unrelated to intrasac pressure.

Despite apparent complete aneurysm exclusion, endotension-associated aneurysm expansion is a clear failure of endoluminal repair. In the absence of an identifiable source of maintained pressurization, however, no endovascular or minimally invasive treatment options exist. In this setting, we recommend multimodality evaluation with CT, CDU, and angiography to maximize the detection of any endoleaks, including characterization of the source and direction of any perigraft flow detected. If aneurysm rupture is to be prevented, close CT scan monitoring and a low threshold for conversion to open repair are essential. We have not found the accuracy and reproducibility of CDU for aneurysm size determinations to be sufficiently high to rely solely on this diagnostic modality for postoperative endograft surveillance, particularly in patients whose aneurysms appear to be expanding.

V. THE SPRINGFIELD EXPERIENCE

An endograft program was initiated at Southern Illinois University School of Medicine/Memorial Medical Center in 1997 as part of the multicenter phase II and III investigational trial of the AneuRx endograft system (Medtronic/AVE Inc., Santa Rosa, CA). The program has expanded to include three other investigational devices—Excluder (WL Gore and Associates Inc., Flagstaff, AZ), AneuRx AUI (Medtronic/AVE Inc., Santa Rosa, CA), and Power Link System (Endologix Inc., Irvine, CA)—as well as the commercially available Ancure device (Guidant Cardiac and Vascular Division, Menlo Park, CA).

Since June 1997, 176 patients had undergone endograft repair of infrarenal aortic aneurysms. There were 20 women and 156 men, with a mean age of 73.5. The mean follow-up period was 21.3 months. In 175 cases an endograft was successfully deployed, while in one patient it became apparent during the early stages of endograft deployment that secure proximal fixation would not be achieved, leading to extraction of the device, procedure termination, and open surgical repair 2 months later. There were no immediate or early conversions, but two patients died within 30 days, for a procedural mortality rate of 1.1%. While there have been no known postoperative aneurysm ruptures, there have been 16 deaths during the follow-up period, 14 of which were definitively unrelated to the procedure. The cause of death is uncertain in the other 2 patients, but aneurysm rupture is not suspected.

A. Primary Endoleaks

At discharge 42 patients had a detectable endoleak. One patient died of unknown causes prior to the 1-month CT scan, and 2 patients refused any postoperative follow-up. Of the of the remaining 39 patients with primary endoleaks and CT scan follow-up, 17 endoleaks were still present at 1 month and 13 at 3 months. Thus, 62% of the primary endoleaks detected at discharge were known to have spontaneously resolved by 3 months. The primary endoleak rate (by actuarial life-table) for the entire series was 24% at discharge, 9.8% at 1 month, and 7.7% at 3 months. In the 13 patients with persistent (>3 months) primary endoleaks, angiography revealed 10 type II endoleaks (8 ilio-lumbar and 2 mesenteric), one distal type I endoleak, and one type III endoleak, and in one patient no endoleak could be demonstrated (indeterminate). Two of the patients died of unrelated causes prior to any intervention, and one type II endoleak resolved spontaneously.

The distal type I endoleak originated from the left common iliac attachment site and was successfully treated by coil embolization of the perigraft channel and outflow lumbar artery (Fig. 4). The type III endoleak originated from an iliac-limb component junction and was successfully sealed by deployment of an additional endograft component. Coil embolization of type II endoleaks was attempted nine times in six patients. While satisfactory deployment of coils at the endoleak site was successful in 8 of the 9 attempts, exclusion of the aneurysm sac was achieved in only four patients. One patient, in which embolization failed, is therapeutically anticoagulated with coumadin for atrial fibrillation and demonstrates continued patency of the IMA and the mesenteric type II endoleak despite multiple coils packed in the proximal IMA. The other patient in whom embolization failed has a persistent ilio-lumbar type II endoleak despite two technically successful embolizations. Repeat embolization is planned for both patients. The aneurysm diameter in the patient with an indeterminate endoleak has remained unchanged for 18 months.

B. Secondary Endoleaks

To date, secondary endoleaks have been detected in 14 patients, 6 first being detected at one month, 2 at 6 months, 4 at 12 months, and 2 at 24 months of follow-up. Four of the leaks detected at one month spontaneously resolved by 3 months. An additional small endoleak that developed late also resolved prior to angiography. In the remaining 9 patients, angiography revealed 3 type II endoleaks (all ilio-lumbar), 2 type III endoleaks, one type I endoleak, 2 indeterminate endoleaks, and angiography is pending in one patient.

Both late type III endoleaks resulted from separation of the main body component of the endograft from a proximal aortic extender component. In one patient the aneurysm was successfully excluded by bridging the defect with a custom tube graft component, and a similar procedure is scheduled for the other. In one patient with a type II endoleak coil embolization was successful, and in another embolization is planned. The remaining patient with a small type II endoleak is being followed and has not shown evidence of aneurysm enlargement on follow-up CT scans. The patient with the secondary type I endoleak underwent successful open surgical repair. This endoleak, first detected at 24 months postendograft, resulted from distal migration of the endograft nearly out of the aneurysm neck caused by an extreme conformation change in the aneurysm itself.

C. Endotension

Five patients have experienced an increase in aneurysm diameter of greater than 0.3 cm without a detectable endoleak (endotension). Four of these patients with modest (<0.6 mm) diameter increases are being followed closely. The remaining patient underwent successful open repair following an increase in the size of the aneurysm from 5.8 to 7.1 cm over an 18-month period. At operation the aneurysm sac was pulsatile, and pressure measurements made by direct puncture without cross-clamping revealed a dampened arterial waveform (pulse pressure) with a systemic mean pressure. Interestingly, blood flow was not detected in the aneurysm sac by intraoperative CDU, nor was any fresh or subacute thrombus or branch vessel bleeding encountered upon opening the unclamped aneurysm. All attachment sites were well incorporated into the vessel wall and hemostatic. After some manipulation of the endograft, however, a small amount of bleeding was noted from the region a suture hole in the graft fabric. While we cannot be certain that this was the source of the endotension present in this patient, it does suggest that such small manufacturing-process fabric defects may behave differently in an endograft and the milieu of an excluded aneurysm than was anticipated based on needle punctures in surgically implanted grafts.

D. Early Versus Late Endoleaks

As noted above, all early endoleaks in our series (i.e., all primary endoleaks and those secondary endoleaks detected at one month) were followed for at least 3 months without intervention. Most of these early endoleaks resolved spontaneously. Conversely, of the 21 patients with late endoleaks (i.e., persistent primary and secondary endoleaks detected at or beyond 3 months of follow-up), spontaneous resolution occurred in only 14%. The majority (62%) of late endoleaks were type II, and of those the ilio-lumbar type predominated (85%). To date, secondary endovascular interventions for late endoleaks for late endoleaks have been successful in excluding the aneurysm sac in 8 of the 10 patients so treated, and one patient has undergone conversion to open repair.

VI. CONCLUSION

Endoluminal repair of infrarenal abdominal aortic aneurysms has gained general acceptance and increasing popularity due to the unequivocal benefits of a short hospital stay, rapid recovery, excellent short-term effectiveness, and low rates of serous complications and mortality. Long-term success of endograft repair ultimately depends upon the prevention of continued aneurysm expansion and subsequent rupture. Achieving this goal will rely on a clearer understanding of the hemodynamics, natural history, accurate diagnosis, and appropriate treatment of postoperative endoleak and endotension. Furthermore, less invasive means of follow-up surveillance and, better yet, minimally invasive mechanisms to measure intrasac pressure will need to be developed for this technology to truly realize all of its purported benefits and gain widespread acceptance among patients, physicians, regulatory agencies, and the medical insurance industry.

REFERENCES

1. White GH, Yu W, May J. Endoleak—a proposed new terminology to describe incomplete aneurysm exclusion by an endoluminal graft. J Endovasc Surg 1996; 3:124–125.

2. White GH, May J, Petrasek P, Waugh R, Stephen M, Harris J. Endotension: an explanation for continued AAA growth after successful endoluminal repair. J Endovasc Surg 1999; 6:308–315.

3. Gilling-Smith GL, Martin J, Sudhindran S, et al. Freedom from endoleak after endovascular aneurysm repair does not equal treatment success. Eur J Vasc Endovasc Surg 2000; 19:421–425.

4. Schunn CD, Krauss M, Heilberger P, Ritter W, Raithel D. Aortic aneurysm size and graft behavior after endovascular stent-grafting: clinical experiences and observations over 3 years. J Endovasc Ther 2000; 7:167–176.

5. Ahn SS, Rutherford RB, Johnston KW, et al. Reporting standards for infrarenal endovascular abdominal aortic aneurysm repair. J Vasc Surg 1997; 25:405–410.

6. Cuypers P, Buth J, Harris PL, Gevers E, Lahey R. Realistic expectations for patients with stent-graft treatment of abdominal aortic aneurysms. Results of a European multicentre registry. Eur J Vasc Endovasc Surg 1999; 17:507–516.

7. Harris PL, Vallabhaneni SR, Desgranges P, Becquemin JP, Van Marrewijk C, Laheij RJ. Incidence and risk factors of late rupture, conversion, and death after endovascular repair of infrarenal aortic aneurysms: the EUROSTAR experience. J Vasc Surg 2000; 32:739–749.

8. Zarins CK, White RA, Hodgson KJ, Schwarten D, Fogarty TJ. Endoleak as a predictor of outcome after endovascular aneurysm repair: AneuRx multicenter clinical trial. J Vasc Surg 2000; 32:90–107.

9. Zarins CK, White RA, Moll FL, et al. The AneuRx stent graft: four-year results and world-wide experience 2000. J Vasc Surg 2001; 33:S135–S145.

10. Wolf YG, Johnson BL, Hill BB, Rubin GD, Fogarty TJ, Zarins CK. Duplex ultrasound scanning versus computed tomographic angiography for postoperative evaluation of endovascular abdominal aortic aneurysm repair. J Vasc Surg 2000; 32:1142–1148.

11. Zannetti S, De Rango P, Parente B, et al. Role of duplex scan in endoleak detection after endoluminal abdominal aortic aneurysm repair. Eur J Vasc Endovasc Surg 2000; 19:531–535.

12. Sato DT, Goff CD, Gregory RT, et al. Endoleak after aortic stent graft repair: diagnosis by color duplex ultrasound scan versus computed tomography scan. J Vasc Surg 1998; 28:657–663.

13. McWilliams RG, Martin J, White D, et al. Use of contrast-enhanced ultrasound in follow-up after endovascular aortic aneurysm repair. J Vasc Interv Radiol 1999; 10:1107–1114.

14. D'Audiffret A, Desgranges P, Kobeiter DH, Becquemin JP. Follow-up evaluation of endoluminally treated abdominal aortic aneurysms with duplex ultrasonography: validation with computed tomography. J Vasc Surg 2001; 33:42–50.

15. Karch LA, Henretta JP, Hodgson KJ, et al. Algorithm for the diagnosis and treatment of endoleaks. Am J Surg 1999; 178:225–231.

16. Albertini J, Kalliafas S, Travis S, et al. Anatomical risk factors for proximal perigraft endoleak and graft migration following endovascular repair of abdominal aortic aneurysms. Eur J Vasc Endovasc Surg 2000; 19:308–312.

17. Greenberg R, Fairman R, Srivastava S, Criado F, Green R. Endovascular grafting in patients with short proximal necks: an analysis of short-term results. Cardiovasc Surg 2000; 8:350–354.

18. Matsumura JS, Chaikof EL. Continued expansion of aortic necks after endovascular repair of abdominal aortic aneurysms. EVT Investigators. EndoVascular Technologies, Inc. J Vasc Surg 1998; 28:422–431.

19. Amesur NB, Zajko AB, Orons PD, Makaroun MS. Embolotherapy of persistent endoleaks after endovascular repair of abdominal aortic aneurysm with the ancure-endovascular technologies endograft system. J Vasc Interv Radiol 1999; 10:1175–1182.

20. Zarins CK, White RA, Fogarty TJ. Aneurysm rupture after endovascular repair using the AneuRx stent graft. J Vasc Surg 2000; 31:960–970.

21. Karch LA, Hodgson KJ, Mattos MA, Bohannon WT, Ramsey DE, McLafferty RB. Management of ectatic, nonaneurysmal iliac arteries during endoluminal aortic aneurysm repair. J Vasc Surg 2001; 33:S33–S38.

22. Baum RA, Carpenter JP, Tuite CM, et al. Diagnosis and treatment of inferior mesenteric arterial endoleaks after endovascular repair of abdominal aortic aneurysms. Radiology 2000; 215:409–413.

23. Puech-Leao P. Banding of the common iliac artery: an expedient in endoluminal correction of aortoiliac aneurysms. J Vasc Surg 2000; 32:1232–1234.

24. Fan CM, Rafferty EA, Geller SC, et al. Endovascular stent-graft in abdominal aortic aneurysms: the relationship between patent vessels that arise from the aneurysmal sac and early endoleak. Radiology 2001; 218:176–182.

25. Velazquez OC, Baum RA, Carpenter JP, et al. Relationship between preoperative patency of the inferior mesenteric artery and subsequent occurrence of type II endoleak in patients undergoing endovascular repair of abdominal aortic aneurysms. J Vasc Surg 2000; 32:777–788.

26. Walker SR, Halliday K, Yusuf SW, et al. A study on the patency of the inferior mesenteric and lumbar arteries in the incidence of endoleak following endovascular repair of infra-renal aortic aneurysms. Clin Radiol 1998; 53:593–595.

27. White RA, Donayre C, Walot I, Stewart M. Abdominal aortic aneurysm rupture following endoluminal graft deployment: report of a predictable event. J Endovasc Ther 2000; 7:257–262.

28. Schurink GW, Aarts NJ, Van Baalen JM, Kool LJ, Van Bockel JH. Experimental study of the influence of endoleak size on pressure in the aneurysm sac and the consequences of thrombosis. Br J Surg 2000; 87:71–78.

29. Baum RA, Carpenter JP, Cope C, et al. Aneurysm sac pressure measurements after endovascular repair of abdominal aortic aneurysms. J Vasc Surg 2001; 33:32–41.

30. van Schie G, Sieunarine K, Holt M, et al. Successful embolization of persistent endoleak from a patent inferior mesenteric artery. J Endovasc Surg 1997; 4:312–315.

31. Gorich J, Rilinger N, Sokiranski R, et al. Embolization of type II endoleaks fed by the inferior mesenteric artery: using the superior mesenteric artery approach. J Endovasc Ther 2000; 7:297–301.

32. Erims C, Kramer S, Tomczak R, et al. Does successful embolization of endoleaks lead to aneurysm sac shrinkage. J Endovasc Ther 2000; 7:441–445.

33. Marty B, Sanchez LA, Ohki T, et al. Endoleak after endovascular graft repair of experimental aortic aneurysms: Does coil embolization with angiographic "seal" lower intraaneurysmal pressure? J Vasc Surg 1998; 27:454–462.

34. van Den Berg JC, Nolthenius RP, Casparie JW, Moll FL. CT-Guided thrombin injection into aneurysm sac in a patient with endoleak after endovascular abdominal aortic aneurysm repair. Am J Roentgenol 2000; 175:1649–1651.

35. Wisselink W, Cuesta MA, Berends FJ, van den Berg FG, Rauwerda JA. Retroperitoneal endoscopic ligation of lumbar and inferior mesenteric arteries as a treatment of persistent endoleak after endoluminal aortic aneurysm repair. J Vasc Surg 2000; 31:1240–1244.

36. Walker SR, Macierewicz J, Hopkinson BR. Endovascular AAA repair: prevention of side branch endoleaks with thrombogenic sponge. J Endovasc Surg 1999; 6:350–353.

37. Midorikawa H, Hoshino S, Iwaya F, Igari T. Graft-wall endoleak 18 months after successful endoluminal AAA repair. J Endovasc Surg 1999; 6:251–255.

38. Holzenbein TJ, Kretschmer G, Thurnher S, et al. Midterm durability of abdominal aortic aneurysm endograft repair: A word of caution. J Vasc Surg 2001; 33:S46–S54.

39. White GH, May J. How should endotension be defined? History of a concept and evolution of a new term. J Endovasc Ther 2000; 7:435–438.

40. Gilling-Smith G, Harris PL, McWilliams RG. How should endotension be defined? J Endovasc Ther 2000; 7:439–440.

41. Fisher RK, Brennan JA, Gilling-Smith GL, Harris PL. Continued sac expansion in the absence of a demonstrable endoleak is an indication for secondary intervention. Eur J Vasc Endovasc Surg 2000; 20:96–98.

15

The Nottingham Perspective with Endoleaks and Endotension: Current Problems and Future Strategies

Robert J. Hinchliffe
University Hospital, Nottingham, England

Brian R. Hopkinson
University of Nottingham and University Hospital, Nottingham, England

I. INTRODUCTION

The early enthusiasm for endovascular repair of abdominal aortic aneurysm has been tempered by sobering reports of aneurysm rupture (1). The purpose of operating on abdominal aortic aneurysm (AAA) is to prevent rupture. We must not lose sight of this fact by becoming distracted with surrogate endpoints such as endoleak. The term endoleak was first coined in 1998 by White and colleagues (2,3) to describe "a condition associated with endoluminal vascular grafts, defined by the presence of blood flow outside the lumen of the endoluminal graft, but within an aneurysm sac or an adjacent vascular segment being treated by the graft."

   Endoleak was noted relatively early in the overall experience of endovascular aneurysm surgery and subsequent reports (4) confirmed that this new terminology could reliably predict outcome. It has also become an important consideration because of reports of its association with aneurysm expansion and rupture. However, more recent reports, such as those from Gilling-Smith et al. (5), Lee et al. (6), and Rhee et al. (7) have refuted this suggestion.

The relevance of an endoleak to the patient's well-being has been further brought into question by reports of aneurysm rupture with no detectable endoleak (8) and in whom the aneurysm sac is shrinking (9).

Unfortunately, the growing burden of evidence has declared that the absence or presence of endoleak cannot predict current or long-term success of an endovascular graft. It was hoped by all in endovascular surgery that the presence or absence of endoleak would correlate directly with the outcome of EVAR, but this is simply not the case. Unfortunately the success of EVAR is more complex than was first realized. Why, therefore, is the term endoleak important, and why is it still widely used?

We maintain that endoleak is a valuable classification and will remain so in the future. In the future, though, it is hoped other more specific parameters may be identified which accurately predict outcome. One of these parameters may include intrasac pressure.

Endoleak may currently be a reliable predictor of secondary intervention requirements. Unfortunately, secondary intervention is surgeon dependent. In most cases it is not known whether these procedures will prevent future morbidity or death. Therefore, unnecessary procedures may be being performed.

It is worthwhile looking at the factors associated with aneurysm rupture de novo. Factors relating to rupture have been investigated in numerous studies. There is little doubt that size is probably the most important determinant of risk of rupture (10). Other risk factors include hypertension, chronic respiratory disease, and smoking (10a,11,12). Both hypertension and chronic respiratory disease appear to be plausible factors. Hypertension probably affects the aneurysm according to the principles of Laplace's law. It is assumed that patients with chronic respiratory disease have increased circulating levels of proteases capable of damaging the aneurysmal wall. Otherwise predicting which aneurysm will rupture is difficult. The reason why one aneurysm ruptures at 5 cm and another at 6 cm is not fully understood. Theories including the ratio of aneurysm diameter to normal aorta have some supporters but have little hard evidence. More complex assessment of aneurysms with mechanical models has been performed, but we have gained little further insight. There are few accurate predictors of aneurysm rupture other than absolute size and possibly asymmetry (13).

The difficulty of identifying predictive factors of de novo rupture of atherosclerotic aneurysms is mirrored in endovascular repair. Patients following open repair have only very small risk of rupture and this is generally related to specific factors such as pseudoaneurysm formation or infection.

The classification of endoleak poses a number of problems not least that each type carries a different prognosis. Unfortunately, and more confusing still, is that there may be variable behavior within each group.

II. TYPE I ENDOLEAK

Type I endoleaks occur after 0–10% of endovascular aortic aneurysm repairs (EVARs). In general we have found that our type I endoleak rate has fallen with a greater understanding of the principles of successful endovascular surgery. Essentially we believe that this complication of EVAR (in the case of primary endoleak, i.e., occurring within 30 days of the procedure) is due to either bad preoperative planning or bad deployment or both in combination. The improvements in preoperative imaging, the understanding of aneurysm morphology, and the recognition of the requirement for oversizing combined with increasing technical expertise have reduced this complication in our institution.

Secondary development (occurring outside the 30-day perioperative period) of type I endoleak may be related to any of the above factors but can also result from non–operator-dependent factors. Essentially, graft migration with/without changing aneurysm morphology and rarely the reopening of a thrombosed channel may cause secondary endoleak (14). Supra-renal stents may prevent graft migration, but the changing morphology of the aneurysm sac following EVAR is complex and may be dependent on the type of stent-graft employed (15) as well as the preoperative morphology [such as heavy circumferential calcium which has been associated with inhibition of sac shrinkage (7)]. There is certainly conflicting evidence regarding the change of aneurysm morphology following both EVAR and open repair. On balance there appears to be some neck dilatation following EVAR and open repair (16,17). The neck expansion has major implications for endografts. Continued neck expansion may predispose to graft migration and endoleak. Unfortunately, a successful repair does not protect the graft from complications, indeed, longitudinal shrinkage of a successfully excluded sac may precipitate graft-limb dislocation (18).

There seems little doubt that type I endoleak is associated with subsequent rupture of the aneurysm sac (19). It is not clear why these endoleaks are particularly dangerous, though direct transmission of pulse pressure must have a role. Our early experience with ruptured AAA repair found proximal perigraft leaks to be universally fatal, most probably due to direct and continued blood loss into the ruptured sac. We did not observe this problem with patent side branch vessels.

Our management of patients with type I endoleak is aggressive. We believe that all these patients are still at risk of rupture. These endoleaks rarely seal spontaneously (20). Therefore, all patients in our institution who have a perigraft leak on completion angiography have corrective treatment before leaving the operating theater.

Patients developing secondary type I leaks invariably require treatment. The treatment depends upon the underlying cause and may involve endovascular or open techniques. The use of packing or embolizing materials has proven disappointing in this group, in our experience. We would not use these methods for proximal type I leak, preferring instead to treat the underlying lesion [supported by the fact that type I endoleaks are the most common indication for transabdominal secondary intervention (19)].

III. TYPE II ENDOLEAK

The accepted type II endoleak rate is in the order of 10–25%, our figures being slightly lower than reported series at 9% (21,22). The etiology of type II endoleak is retrograde perfusion of the aneurysm sac, most often from the lumbar or inferior mesenteric arteries (IMA) (23,24) (Fig. 1). Velazquez and colleagues have demonstrated that thrombosed inferior mesenteric arteries do not cause leaks but that one quarter of patent IMAs will subsequently perfuse the sac and may be involved in a "circuit" with patent lumbar arteries (27).

It has been recognized from the early days of EVAR that type II endoleaks generally run a much more benign course when compared with type I endoleak (46). The natural history of type II endoleaks is such that they, on the whole, do not cause increasing size of the aneurysm sac (25). Somewhere in the region of two thirds will spontaneously thrombose in the perioperative period.

Unfortunately, there appear to be no identifiable factors that strongly predispose to type II endoleak (26). The analysis of data provided by the EUROSTAR registry (19) suggested the number and size of preoperative feeding vessels and the Stentor device had statistically significant associations, but this has not been echoed by other authors (24,27). As a result these authors recommended that preoperative treatment of IMAs or lumbar arteries should not be undertaken.

The exact implications of type II endoleak are not yet fully understood. Useful parallels may be drawn from open surgery. Resnikoff's experience with nonresective treatment of AAA sheds some light on the issue of perigraft flow secondary to patent collateral vessels (28). Seventeen patients out of a

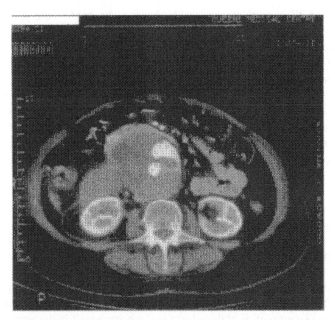

Figure 1. Patent inferior mesenteric artery producing a type II endoleak following endovascular repair of a ruptured abdominal aortic aneurysm.

total of 831 required intraoperative ligation of collaterals. During a follow-up of between 5 and 103 months, a further 17 (2%) aneurysm sacs remained patent on duplex scanning. Fourteen of these patients received treatment; 4 of these were for sac rupture and 3 for pain. Patients with rupture exhibited some consistent findings on prerupture duplex scanning, namely no shrinkage of the aneurysm sac, positive wall motion with respect to the cardiac cycle, and finally flow within the sac. These factors have also been associated with endoleaks in EVAR (29,30).

A number of important factors come out of this valuable paper. First, it has confirmed our findings that retroleak may occur sometime after the operation despite apparent successful ligation either pre- or intraoperatively. Second, it emphasizes a number of important investigative findings that may predict rupture. Third, it demonstrates the importance of regular follow-up of excluded aneurysms to prevent rupture. And finally, it confirms that type II endoleak may cause rupture. Systemic pressure within the aneurysm sac of a patient with type II endoleak has been demonstrated on a number of occasions both in vitro (31) and in vivo (32). Quite why the majority of these patients appear to have a favorable outcome despite exposing their aneurysm sacs to systemic pressures is unknown. It does not appear to be related to the presence of a pulsatile waveform as these were recorded in all patients with both types (I and II) of endoleak in recent publications by Baum et al. (33,34).

Despite early reports of the benign nature of type II leaks, there is some weight of data emerging that challenges this belief. As stated above the measurement of systemic pressures combined with pulsatile waveforms is rather disconcerting. Arko has recorded in his experience that chronic type II endoleaks tended to increase both aneurysm sac diameter and volume, both of which may be regarded as parameters of unsuccessful treatment (35). A rather worrying tendency implicating type II endoleaks with sac rupture has emerged from the EUROSTAR database (19). And finally, pressure transmission to the sac has also been noted in type II endoleaks that have sealed spontaneously, the pressure presumably being transmitted via thrombus (which may also have major implications for the treatment of these endoleaks by inducing thrombosis via embolization) (36).

Treatment for this type of endoleak is controversial. Preoperative treatment has been suggested, though we would prefer not to undertake it because a great proportion of these leaks seal spontaneously in the perioperative period. Some authors, including Baum, take an aggressive approach to their treatment, stating the transmission of systemic pressure as a reason to indicate their potential to cause rupture. Although type II endoleaks undoubtedly transmit pressure themselves, it is not obvious whether the pressure in the endoleak channel is reflected by changes in the rest of the aneurysm sac and, more importantly, on the wall of the sac. [Baum et al. (33) claim that pressure within the wall thrombus does mimic that in the endoleak. Other studies recording pressures did not do so within various parts of the aneurysm sac.] Whatever the pressure finding, the majority of type II endoleaks appear to seal spontaneously and subsequently appear to cause no harm.

Treatment of type II endoleaks postoperatively has largely been performed by embolization techniques. The access used for embolization has varied and included a direct translumbar approach and a number of different endovascular methods. Using these methods, the majority of endoleaks may be treated successfully. Access tends to be the factor resulting in treatment failure rather than the procedure of embolization itself (37). Unfortunately, despite the apparent success of embolization in the short term, there are insufficient data to assess long-term outcome. More specifically it is not yet clear whether embolized type II leaks behave any differently from spontaneously thrombosed leaks (38).

Another approach to the management of type II endoleak is to prevent them at the time of operation. We prefer to try and prevent type II endoleaks intraoperatively. Passing sizable catheters directly into the aneurysm sac in the presence of systemic pressures, disturbing iliac limbs, and simple angiography all carry a degree of risk, whereas our method avoids or minimizes such problems. Intraoperative aneurysm packing involves inserting thrombogenic sponge directly in to the aneurysm sac following a "sacogram" to identify any patent collateral branches (39) (Figs. 2 and 3). Using this method we have reduced our type II endoleaks considerably, with reduction maintained at both 1- (40) and 2-year (41) follow-up. (Original preaneurysm packing type II leak rate was 9%. It is now reduced to 1.3% at 2 years follow-up.) Aneurysm packing is becoming more widespread, and we are aware that it has been used by Parodi and others. Indeed, the use of aneurysm packing in an attempt to reduce wall stress is far from being a new technique, having been used by Moore in 1864 (42) and more recently by Peacock in the 1960s. Essentially in the open case the packing was employed in an attempt to reduce wall stress. In EVAR its use is primarily in the prevention of leaks or in the induction of collateral vessel thrombosis. Some centers are employing other packing materials, including onyx® (43). This use of onyx has reduced sac pressures to near zero in type 2 leaks but has not been attempted for attachment site leaks.

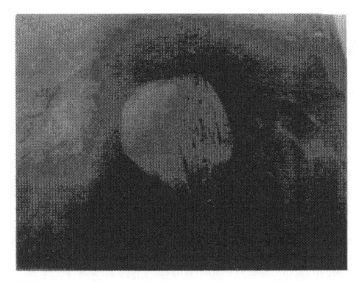

Figure 2.   Negative intraoperative sacogram ("aneurysmogram").

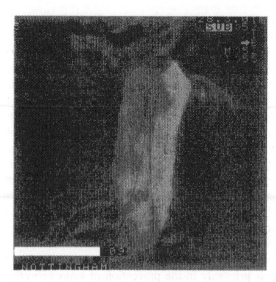

Figure 3.   Positive intraoperative sacogram that identifies an accessory renal artery not identified preoperatively.

Aneurysm packing with nonabsorbable materials has introduced a new concept to aneurysm surgery, which is one of maintaining the sac postoperatively, as a solid structure, rather than the current quest for its obliteration (43).

IV. TYPE III ENDOLEAK

This type of endoleak invariably requires treatment and can be attributed to graft failure (44). Type III endoleak has been associated with rupture of the sac as reported by the EUROSTAR collaborators (19) and others (45). It has been consistently associated with a number of graft designs, some of which have been withdrawn from commercial use. The type of graft failure has been variable but has included modular limb dislocation and direct damage of graft material by a stented exoskelelton. Patients with type III endoleak may be suddenly exposed to systemic pulsatile pressure. It remains to be seen whether patients whose aneurysm sac has shrunken following treatment will be more susceptible to rupture when compared to early type III leak where the sac has not atrophied.

V. TYPE IV ENDOLEAK

Type IV endoleaks are seen as a consequence of a desire to scale down the size of introduction sheaths by reducing the graft-wall thickness. The AneuRx graft is the classical thin-walled graft. It characteristically produces a "blush" of contrast on a CTA performed in the first week (46). Fortunately, the natural history of these "leaks" is to seal spontaneously, and intervention has rarely been required. The long-term durability of these grafts has been brought into question by the problems associated with graft porosity and failure. The durability of thin-walled grafts remains undetermined.

VI. ENDOTENSION

The term endotension was introduced following the observation that a number of aneurysm sacs were expanding despite the apparent absence of endoleak (47). This observation may have been explained by the quality of diagnostic imaging in some cases (i.e., missed endoleaks), or by the concept of intermittent endoleak described by Gilling-Smith et al.(48). This group also subclassified endotension into grades 1 (high flow), 2 (low flow), and 3 (absence of flow).

The observation of pressure transmission via thrombus is not limited to EVAR. Following aorto-bifemoral bypass, a patient may exsanguinate from an aortic stump ruptured despite the presence of thrombus extending up to the renal arteries. It was also appreciated that patients with an occluded aortic aneurysm may still rupture (Figs. 4, 5).

Although it is widely regarded that size of endoleak does not affect the size of pressure transmission (49), recent evidence from Ohki and colleagues presented at the international symposium of critical issues in endovascular aneurysm surgery has indicated that "short, fat" thrombosed endoleaks may well transmit a greater pressure than "long, thin" ones, which may well explain why pressure via a type I endoleak, even if thrombosed, is dangerous. [The presence of thrombosed endoleak channels were highlighted by cases such as that described by Resh et al. A proximal endoleak channel declared itself following thrombolysis of an occluded stent-graft, the patient subsequently died from aneurysm rupture, which was attributed to the thrombolysis of the thrombosed endoleak endoleak channel (50).]

Currently we have the means to measure sac pressures in short periods. Several authors have shown a reduction of sac pressures in successfully excluded aneurysm sacs (51). Others have also shown that the pressure does not drop in the presence of endoleaks (52,53). Unfortunately, we cannot measure pressure over longer time periods. It would be advantageous to understand pressure variation in response to the development of an endoleak or, conversely, the effects of endoleak treatment in the long term. The current pressure transducers available are also flawed by their size and requirement for wires, which may kink or allow flow of blood into the aneurysm sac, thus producing misleading results.

It was hoped that pressure measurement would be able to predict which endoleaks required treatment. Unfortunately, it appears that the majority of patients undergoing pressure measurement of their aneurysm sacs during intervention for endoleak express systemic pulsatile pressures. Therefore, the level of pressure per se may not be a useful indicator of a successful endoleak treatment/aneurysm exclusion, but it may be a useful tool if the pressure change over time can be recorded. Further investigation and an implantable

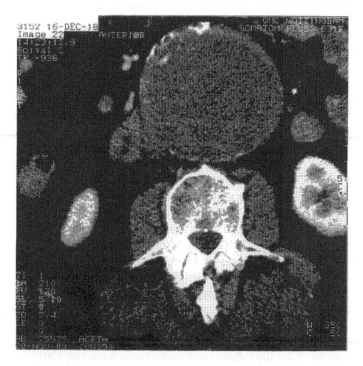

Figure 4. Thrombosed AAA. An infrarenal stent-graft had been deployed in this patient 6 years previously. The stent-graft subsequently migrated. The patient was too frail to consider further intervention and later presented with a ruptured AAA (see Fig. 5).

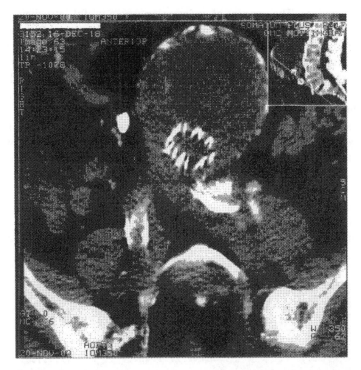

Figure 4. Continued.

pressure transducer might clear up some of the questions that remain, specifically how pressure varies within different areas of the sac, changes of pressure over time, and the effect of intervention on pressure. Assessing aneurysm size is a reliable detector of outcome and may be a potent indicator of continued aneurysm exclusion (54). Unfortunately, time is taken for the aneurysm sac to alter size (55) (any real change may take up to one year to appear), and it may therefore lag any real change in status of the patient. And, interestingly, as discussed previously, aneurysm shrinkage may not occur despite apparently successful treatment (56).

VII. CONCLUSIONS

The current classification of endoleak is a useful one, however, it does not identify those patients who necessarily require secondary intervention to prevent rupture. The concept of endotension was a useful introduction as it sought to identify those at increased risk of aneurysm rupture. Patients with endotension are subject to raised pressures within the aneurysm sac, which may or may not be due to an identified endoleak. The terminology has therefore moved away from the observation that the patient simply has an endoleak or not. It has reinforced the importance of measuring intrasac pressures.

Although it is widely accepted that persisitent pressurization of the aneurysm sac may lead to rupture, many questions remain unanswered. Importantly, what levels of pressure and what type of pressure waveforms put the aneurysm sac at risk of expansion and rupture? Indeed it is unlikely that these parameters will be the same between patients, just as aneurysms rupture at different diameters.

Our major problem at the moment is the type II endoleak. It has been recognized by most investigators to have a benign course, but there have been

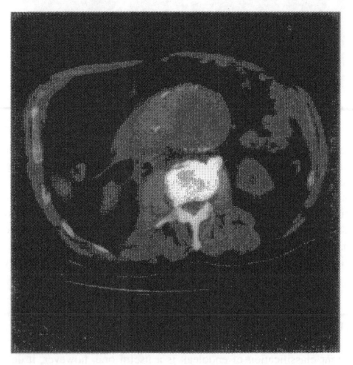

Figure 5. Endotension: rupture of the aneurysm in the patient shown in Figure 4.

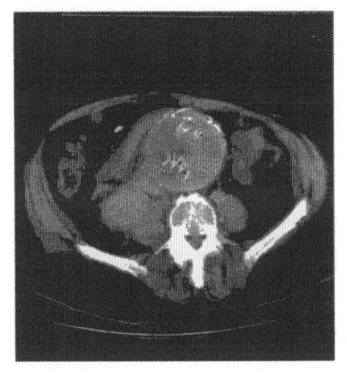

Figure 5. Continued.

reports of increasing aneurysm size and rupture. How do we identify dangerous type II leaks? Is simple embolization sufficient to satisfactorily reduce pressure and prevent rupture in the long term? Unfortunately, pressure studies on type II leaks have revealed systemic and pulsatile pressures in most, therefore, why are they behaving differently from type I leaks? It may be that we are simply observing the natural history of untreated AAA in patients with type II endoleak. Further study of intrasac pressure is required to fully understand the implications of this complication.

It is clear from the literature that patients who have undergone endovascular grafting require regular assessment of their aneurysm and endograft. The current "best buy" modality of imaging appears to be spiral CTA, but duplex assessment may have a role.

The endovascular surgeon wants to know which of his patients are at risk of rupture. The answer is that all are potentially at risk of rupture, and therefore all currently require follow-up. However, there are certain high-risk patients, some of whom have endoleak. There is good evidence that both type I and type III endoleaks are associated with rupture. Patients with an increasing aneurysm diameter (or volume) despite EVAR have endotension and require further investigation to identify a cause if one is not already apparent. Treatment of these patients is needed as the aneurysm is not excluded from the circulation. Current evidence on type II endoleak is insufficient although it appears safe to simply watch this cohort of patients as long as their aneurysms are not growing.

The final area of concern is the patient in whom the aneurysm sac is static in the absence of endoleak. We simply do not have the information to know whether this patient remains at risk of rupture. Logically it would appear that a patient with a 5.5 cm AAA would maintain the same risk, but this is purely speculative. It is interesting to note that aneurysm sac shrinkage may not occur in the expected fashion in all patients, particularly those with heavy calcification of their aneurysm wall (7). In these patients intervention may not be required.

REFERENCES

1. Lumsden AB, Allen RC, Chaikof EL, et al. Delayed rupture of aortic aneurysms following endovascular stent grafting. Am J Surg 1995; 170:174–178.
2. White GH, May J, Waugh RC, et al. Type 1 and type 2 endoleaks: a more useful classification for reporting results of endoluminal AAA repair (letter). J Endovasc Surg 1998; 5:189–191.
3. White GH, May J, Waugh RC, et al. Type 3 and type 4 endoleak: toward a complete definition of blood flow in the sac after endoluminal AAA repair. J Endovasc Surg 1998; 5:305–309.
4. Matsumara JS, Moore WS. Clinical consequences of periprosthetic leak after endovascular repair of abdominal aortic aneurysm. J Vasc Surg 1998; 27:606–613.
5. Gilling-Smith GL, Martin J, Sudhindran S, et al. Freedom from endoleak after endovascular aneurysm repair does not equal treatment success. Eur J Vasc Endovasc Surg 2000; 19:621–625.
6. Lee WA, Yehuda GW, Fogarty TJ, et al. Does complete aneurysm exclusion ensure long-term success after endovascular repair? J Endovasc Ther 2000; 7:494–500.
7. Rhee RY, Eskandari MK, Zajko AB, et al. Long-term fate of the aneurysmal sac after endoluminal exclusion of abdominal aortic aneurysms. J Vasc Surg 2000; 32:689–696.

8. Torsello GB, Klenk E, Kasprzak B, et al. Rupture of abdominal aortic aneurysm previously treated by endograft stent-graft. J Vasc Surg 1998; 28:184–187.

9. Alimi YS, Chakfe N, Rivoal E, et al. Rupture of an abdominal aortic aneurysm after endovascular graft placement and aneurysm size reduction. J Vasc Surg 1998; 28:178–183.

10. Szilagyi DE, Elliott JP, Smith RF, et al. Clinical fate of the patient with asymptomatic aortic aneurysm and unfit for surgical treatment. Arch Surg 1972; 104:600.

10a. MacSweeney ST, Ellis M, Worrell PC, et al. Smoking and growth rate of small abdominal aortic aneurysms. Lancet 1994; 344:651–652.

11. Cronewett JL, Murphy TF, Zelenock GB, et al. Actuarial analysis of variables associated with rupture of small abdominal aortic aneurysms. Surgery 1995; 98:472.

12. Sterpetti AV, Cavallaro A, Cavallari N, et al. Factors influencing the rupture of abdominal aortic aneurysm. Surg Obstet Gynecol 1991; 173:175.

13. Vorp DA, Raghavan ML, Webster MW. Mechanical wall stress in abdominal aortic aneurysm: Influence of diameter and asymmetry. J Vasc Surg 1998; 27:632.

14. Wever JJ, Blankensteijn JD, Eikelboom BC. Secondary endoleak or missed endoleak? Eur J Vasc Surg 1999; 18:458–460.

15. Singh-Ranger R, Adiseshiah M. Differing morphological changes following endovascular AAA repair using balloon-expandable or self-expandable endografts. J Endovasc Ther 2000; 7:479–485.

16. Matsumara JS, Chaikof EL. Continued expansion of aortic necks after endovascular repair of abdominal aortic aneurysms. J Vasc Surg 1998; 28:422–431.

17. Illig KA, Green RM, Ouriel K, et al. Fate of the proximal aortic cuff: implications for endovascular aneurysm repair. J Vasc Surg 1998; 28:184–187.

18. Harris P, Brennan J, Martin J, et al. Longitudinal aneurysm shrinkage following endovascular aortic aneurysm repair: a source of intermediate and late complications. J Endovasc Surg 1999; 6:11–16.

19. Laheij RJF, Buth J, Harris PL, et al. Need for secondary interventions after endovascular repair of abdominal aortic aneurysms. Intermediate-term follow-up results of a European collaborative registry (EUROSTAR). Br J Surg 2000; 87:1666–1673.

20. May J, White GH, et al. Endovascular treatment of aortic aneurysms. In Rutherfords Vascular Surgery, Cronenwett JL, Ed.; Philadelphia: WB Saunders; 2000:1288.

21. Jacobowitz GR, Rosen RJ, Riles TS. The significance and management of the leaking endograft. Semin Vasc Surg 1999; 12:199–206.

22. White GH, Yu W, May J, et al. Endoleak as a complication of endoluminal grafting of abdominal aortic aneurysms: classification, incidence, diagnosis and management. J Endovasc Surg 1997; 4:152–168.

23. Goodman MA, Lawrence-Brown M, et al. "Retroleak"—retrograde branch filling of the excluded aneurysm (letter). J Endovasc Surg 1998; 5:378.

24. White GH, May J, Waugh RC, et al. Re: "Retroleak"—retrograde branch filling of the excluded aneurysm (letter). J Endovasc Surg 1998; 5:378–379.

25. Resch T, Ivancev K, Lindh M, et al. Persistent collateral perfusion of abdominal aortic aneurysm after endovascular repair does not lead to progressive change in aneurysm diameter. J Vasc Surg 1998; 28:242–249.

26. Walker SR, Halliday K, Yusuf SW, et al. A study on the patency of the inferior mesenteric and lumbar arteries in the incidence of endoleak following endovascular repair of infrarenal aortic aneurysms. Clin Radiol 1998; 53:593–595.

27. Velazquez OC, Baum RA, Carpenter JP, et al. Relationship between preoperative patency of the inferior mesenteric artery and subsequent occurrence of type 2 endoleak in patients undergoing endovascular repair of abdominal aortic aneurysms. J Vasc Surg 2000; 32:777–788.

28. Resnikoff M, Darling RC, Chang BB, et al. Fate of the excluded abdominal aortic aneurysm sac: long-term follow-up of 831 patients. J Vasc Surg 1995; 21:623–634.

29. Malina M, Lanne T, Ivancev K, et al. Reduced pulsatile wall motion of abdominal aortic aneurysms after endovascular repair. J Vasc Surg 1998; 27:624–631.

30. McWilliams R, Martin J, Gould D, et al. Levovist-enhanced ultrasound as the primary follow-up investigation after endovascular aneurysm repair. J Intervent Radiol 1998; 13:146–147.

31. Gilling-Smith GL, Chong CK, How TV, et al. Endovascular repair of abdominal aortic aneurysm: How dangerous are side branch endoleaks? (abstr). J Endovasc Surg 1999; 6:73–123.

32. Gilling-Smith GL, Chong CK, How TV, et al. Endovascular repair of abdominal aortic aneurysm: How dangerous are side branch endoleaks? (abstr). J Endovasc Surg 1999; 6:73–123.

33. Baum RA, Carpenter JP, Cope C, et al. Aneurysm sac pressure measurements after endovascular repair of abdominal aortic aneurysms. J Vasc Surg 2000; 33:32–40.

34. Baum RA, Carpenter JC, Tuite CM, et al. Diagnosis and treatment of inferior mesenteric arterial endoleaks after endovascular repair of abdominal aortic aneurysms. Radiology 2000; 215:409–413.

35. Arko FR, Rubin GD, Johnson BL, et al. Type 2 endoleaks following endovascular repair: preoperative predictors and long-term effects. International Congress 14 on Endovascular Interventions, New York, 2000.

36. Clement Darling R, Ozavath K, Chang BB, et al. The incidence, natural history, and outcome of secondary intervention for persistent collateral flow in the excluded abdominal aortic aneurysm. J Vasc Surg 1999; 30:968–976.

37. Gorich J, Rilinger N, Sokiranski R, et al. Embolization of type 2 endoleaks fed by the inferior mesenteric artery: using the superior mesenteric artery approach. J Endovasc Ther 2000; 7:297–301.

38. Marty B, Sanchez LA, Ohki T, et al. Endoleak after endovascular graft repair of experimental aneurysms: Does coil embolization with angiographic "seal" lower intraaneurysmal pressure? J Vasc Surg 1998; 27:454–461.

39. Walker SR, Macierewicz JA, Hopkinson BR. Endovascular AAA repair: prevention of side branch endoleaks with thrombogenic sponge. J Endovasc Surg 1999; 6:350–353.

40. Lehmann JM, Macierewicz JA, Davidson IR, et al. Prevention of side branch endoleaks with thrombogenic sponge: one year follow-up. J Endovasc Ther 2000; 7:431–433.

41. Hinchliffe RJ, Hopkinson BR. Clinical and experimental evidence of benefits by packing aneurysm sacs following endografting. International Symposium in Critical Issues in Endovascular Aneurysm Surgery, Leiden, Netherlands, February 2001.

42. Keen, WW. Surgery: Its Principles and Practice. WB Saunders: Philadelphia, 1921:216–349.

43. Fry PD, Martin M, Machan L. Endoleaks and the need for a paradigm shift (letter). J Endovasc Ther 2000; 7:521–522.

44. White G, May J, Waugh RC, et al. Type 3 and type 4 endoleak: toward a complete definition of blood flow in the sac after endoluminal repair. J Endovasc Surg 1998; 5:305–309.

45. Maleux G, Rousseau H, Otal P, et al. Modular component separation and reperfusion of abdominal aortic aneurysm sac after endovascular repair of the abdominal aoeric aneurysm: a case report. J Vasc Surg 1998; 28:349–352.

46. Zarins CK, White RA, Schwarten DE, et al. AneuRX stent-graft versus open repair of abdominal aortic aneurysms: multicentre prospective clinical trial. J Vasc Surg 1999; 29:292–308.

47. White GH, May J, Petrasek P, et al. Endotension: an explanation for continued AAA growth after successful endoluminal repair. J Endovasc Surg 1999; 6:308–315.

48. Gilling-Smith GL, Brennan J, Harris P, et al. Endotension after endovascular aneurysm repair: definition, classification, and stratagies for surveillance and intervention. J Endovasc Surg 1999; 6:305–307.

49. Schurink GW, Aarts NJ, Van Baalen JM, et al. Experimental study of the influence of endoleak size on pressure in the aneurysm sac and the consequences of thrombosis. Br J Surg 2000; 87:71–78.

50. Resch T, Lindblad B, Lindh M, et al. Aneurysm expansion and retroperitoneal haematoma after thrombolysis for stent-graft limb occlusion caused by distal endograft migration. J Endovasc Ther 2000; 7:446–450.

51. Chuter T, Ivancev K, Malina M, et al. Aneurysm pressure following endovascular exclusion. Eur J Vasc Endovasc Surg 1997; 13:85–87.

52. Treharne GD, Loftus IM, Thompson MM, et al. Quality control during endovascular aneurysm repair: monitoring aneurismal sac pressure and superficial femoral artery flow velocity. J Endovasc Surg 1999; 6:239–245.

53. Stelter W, Umscheid T, Ziegler P. Three-year experience with modular stent-graft devices for endovascular AAA treatment. J Endovasc Surg 1997; 4:362–369.
54. Broeders IA, Blankensteijn JD, Gvakharia A, et al. The efficacy of transfemoral endovascular aneurysm management: a study on size changes of the abdominal aorta during mid-term follow-up. Eur J Vasc Endovasc Surg 1997; 14:84–90.
55. Wolf YG, Hill BR, Rubin GD, et al. Rate of change in abdominal aortic aneurysm diameter after endovascular repair. J Vasc Surg 2000; 32:108–115.
56. Guident/EVT. Review of the Ancure 2 year clinical data (customer brochure). June 2000.

16

Endoleak Behavior Is Graft Specific

NavYash Gupta and Michel S. Makaroun
*University of Pittsburgh Medical Center and Presbyterian University Hospital,
Pittsburgh, Pennsylvania, U.S.A.*

The past decade has given us the opportunity to accumulate an increasing amount of data relating to the use of endovascular technology for the treatment of abdominal aortic aneurysms (AAA). The devices continue to be refined, and some have become commercially available, allowing for the widespread application of this treatment. Initial clinical trials have reported high success rates for the endovascular exclusion of AAAs (1–4), but the long-term durability and success of endografts remains suspect, as many early and late failures have been reported (5–7).

Perhaps the most concerning of these problems is the persistence of blood flow around the endograft into the aneurysm sac. This phenomenon, termed an endoleak, implies the continued exposure of the aneurysmal sac to systemic arterial pressure. A report from our group during our early experience with coiling of endoleaks made note of the elevated pressures within the aneurysm sac of such patients (8). Others have reported similar findings (9). The clinical significance of such endoleaks, however, remains unsettled, with very divergent opinions. The presence of an endoleak has been regarded by some as a failure of the endovascular procedure (10,11). Others have found that endoleaks detected by contrast enhanced computerized tomography (CT) scans are nonpredictive of the risk of aneurysm rupture and patient survival following endovascular aneurysm repair (3).

The classification of endoleaks into 4 types proposed by White and colleagues (12) has been widely adopted. The various types are separated based on the source of the perigraft flow, and the clinical characteristics of

185

such endoleaks have long been assumed to be dependent, for the most part, on the specific type. Although very useful, this classification system is often imprecise without angiographic examination, and not always predictive of outcome. The clinical behavior of endoleaks has remained quite difficult to predict, even when appropriately classified. Whereas some aneurysms continue to expand and in some cases lead to rupture, others remain stable or may even shrink in size (13–16). Occasionally an aneurysm enlarges without an apparent endoleak, and ruptures have occurred in this situation (17,18). A recent report detailing a significant series of rupture of the AAA after endovascular repair highlighted the importance of proximal sealing of the device in the neck of the aneurysm (19).

In a volume dedicated to endoleaks with many contributors, it is difficult to avoid duplication of information. We will attempt to propose mostly one new concept in this chapter, namely that the clinical behavior of endoleaks is graft specific in several aspects. This is a variable that has been underestimated in the discussion of endoleaks and their treatment and is not reflected in the commonly used White classification. Our large experience with a nonsupported, unibody endograft that differs sharply in design from the majority of stent grafts has led us to observe some differences in the clinical behavior of endoleaks among different grafts. Recognition of these differences among endografts will allow for a better comparison of reports that seem to be contradictory at times.

I. CLINICAL EXPERIENCE

We have used four different systems for the endovascular exclusion of AAA. From February 1996 to February 2001, we repaired 325 AAAs with commercially manufactured systems. Most of our patients (261) were treated with the Ancure endograft system (Guidant Endovascular Solutions, Inc., Menlo Park, CA). Other grafts used were the Excluder (W. L. Gore and Associates, Flagstaff, AZ), the AneuRx (Medtronic, Minneapolis, MN), and the Talent device (World Medical/Medtronic Corp., Sunrise, FL). Our initial experience was part of the multicenter phase II or III evaluation of these grafts with an additional 205 repairs performed since FDA approval of the Ancure and AneuRx endografts in September 1999. All patients underwent an intraoperative angiogram to assess the adequacy of device placement and aneurysmal exclusion. Initial assessment of results was performed within one month on all patients using contrast enhanced CT, duplex scanning, and plain films. A 6-month CT scan was obtained on all phase II patients and all subsequent patients with a recognizable endoleak during the initial assessment. All patients also had yearly evaluations thereafter. Any patient with incomplete exclusion of the AAA on any study within one month of implantation, including the intraoperative completion angiogram, was considered to have an endoleak. Late presence or absence of endoleaks was determined from contrast enhanced CT. In case of renal failure or contrast allergy, duplex scanning was used as the determinant factor.

The records as well as the pre- and postoperative imaging studies of all patients with endoleaks were reviewed. Preoperative variables that were compared between the group of patients that developed endoleaks versus the group that did not included size of the AAA, size of the native artery at the attachment sites, degree of calcification, and mural thrombus. Angulation of the neck was also measured, and the status of preoperative patent branches of the AAA was determined.

II. DIAGNOSIS OF ENDOLEAK TYPE

During the initial phase II and III evaluations of these endografts, we classified the site of the endoleak by information obtained from all three diagnostic modalities used in the immediate postoperative evaluation. This included the intraoperative angiogram, a contrast enhanced CT scan, and duplex ultrasonography, which were performed within a month of endograft placement.

The imprecision of the present classification system is highlighted by the following observation. During our initial experience with 158 patients undergoing endovascular repair of AAA, 11 patients were noted to have persistent endoleak at 6-month follow-up. A group of independent observers at a core laboratory reviewing CT and ultrasound exams on these patients felt that the majority of these endoleaks were type II in nature. However, at the time of angiography, routinely performed for persistent endoleaks, 6 patients were noted to have attachment site endoleaks (type I), 3 were due to reversed flow in the IMA, and one patient had an endoleak due to ilio-lumbar collaterals (type II). One patient demonstrated no evidence of endoleak, and a repeat CT scan showed spontaneous resolution of the endoleak. There was a 6-week delay between the CT scan study showing the endoleak and the arteriogram, and the endoleak presumably sealed in this interim.

The inadequacy of noninvasive modalities to properly diagnose the source of the endoleak has not been properly assessed for many grafts. This finding is definitely true for the Ancure system, and we suspect it is also true for all endografts. Although both CT scanning and ultrasonography significantly aid in the diagnosis of an endoleak, these studies cannot be reliably used to determine the type of endoleak. Hence, we feel that the decision to intervene on a persistent endoleak should not be solely based on a classification of the endoleak by standard CT scanning and duplex scanning, since they can be misleading. The mere presence of a persistent endoleak on either imaging study should encourage further evaluation by angiography to plan further management.

Our current protocol includes an intraoperative angiogram to assess adequacy of device placement and aneurysm exclusion followed by a CT scan performed within the first month of graft placement. If no endoleak is detected on the CT scan, the patients return for an annual exam. Patients noted to have an endoleak return for a 6-month study, and if a persistent endoleak is still detected, further evaluation and aggressive treatment is implemented.

III. INCIDENCE AND TYPE OF ENDOLEAK

Endoleaks have been reported with all systems, but only type I and type II endoleaks have been described with the Ancure system. Device design does play a major role relating to this observation. Type III endoleaks have been noted with modular systems where a disjunction of the overlap zones results in a leak between the parts of the system. In addition, this type of endoleak has been described at stent to graft suture lines in the body of the aneurysm and in association with very thin fabric. The unibody design of the Ancure system and the standard polyester fabric eliminate the possibility of this type of endoleak. Type IV endoleaks have been noted as temporary graft material porosity, which may be related to the thin fabric used in the design of some grafts. Again, this type of endoleak has not been reported with the Ancure system. This illustrates that endoleak sources can be different among grafts.

The incidence of endoleaks may be different among different endografts. In our experience, the total incidence of endoleaks appears to be higher with the Ancure system (up to 38% with our phase II patients) as compared to the Excluder device (20% for phase II patients) (4,8,20).

Although many factors including learning curves and availability of other devices may have played a role in this observation, we believe it to be a true finding. Our endoleak rate with the Ancure system is similar to the rate reported in published data with the EVT device from other centers (21,22), and reported data with newer fully supported rigid or semi-rigid design grafts also suggest a lower early endoleak rate following deployment.

Possible explanation for this difference in observed endoleak rate may again relate to the unsupported unibody design of the Ancure system. A fully supported, more rigid endograft, such as the Excluder device, may allow for better initial apposition over a longer length between the external surface of the graft and the luminal surface of the artery wall. In addition, modular components allow for more intraoperative manipulations to eliminate endoleak sources.

It is hard to predict which patients will have an endoleak. Analysis of our data revealed no difference in aneurysm size, neck diameter, or distal attachment-site diameter between patients with and without endoleaks. The degree of calcification and presence of mural thrombus were also similar between the two groups. The presence or absence, on preoperative angiogram, of large branches such as lumbars, accessory renals, or the IMA did not appear to be predictive of endoleaks.

Neck angulation, however, does appear to play a role in the development of a proximal endoleaks with the Ancure graft (8) and most likely with other endografts. All our patients with endoleaks associated with the proximal attachment system had an angulation of the proximal neck in excess of 35 degrees to the main flow channel of the AAA. The likelihood of developing a proximal attachment system endoleak was 50% if the angle on preoperative angiography exceeded 35 degrees.

Graft configuration also appeared to play a role with the Ancure system. The lowest incidence of endoleak was noted with the "bifurcated" configuration (21%) compared with the "tube" (50%) and the "aorto-iliac" (43%). Comparisons to other endograft systems should then use data from the appropriate configuration to be meaningful.

IV. SPONTANEOUS RESOLUTION

Spontaneous resolution of endoleaks has been well documented in the majority of cases (4,14,21). In our experience, about two thirds of endoleaks can be expected to seal on their own during a 6-month follow-up. Certain endoleaks seem to resolve much more readily than others. This area provides one of the most striking differences among grafts.

The vast majority of our proximal attachment system endoleaks with the Ancure endograft detected intraoperatively stopped spontaneously, a finding quite dissimilar from other systems. Almost all these endoleaks seem to resolve by the first follow-up imaging obtained usually at one month. We feel increasingly confident that type I proximal endoleaks noted at the time of endograft placement with the Ancure system are benign in nature and most will disappear by 1 month (Fig. 1). This cannot be said about a proximal type I endoleak noted with a fully supported graft. Such an endoleak is best treated at the time of graft placement with an extension cuff or some other means rather than being managed expectantly. The difference is probably related to the low radial force of the large Ancure attachment system and the sharp change in rigidity at the transition level to an unsupported graft. This leads sometimes, most notably with angulated necks, to initial incomplete apposition that gradually remodels with time to result in complete exclusion.

The same has not been true for distal type I endoleaks among our Ancure patients (8,23). The documentation of an endoleak at that location is quite common among the persistent endoleaks with the Ancure system in our series. The likelihood that the distal attachment system will seal seems to be less likely over time in ectatic or tortuous iliac arteries. Again, the unsupported

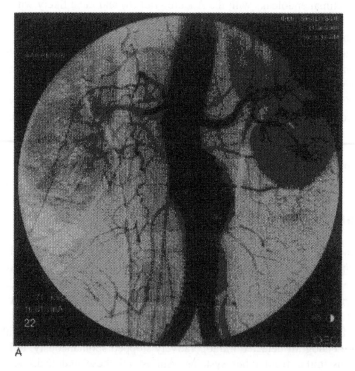

A

Figure 1.   (A) Arteriogram demonstrating a type I proximal endoleak following endovascular repair of an AAA with the Ancure system. (B) CT scan of the same patient performed 2 weeks later shows no evidence of endoleak.

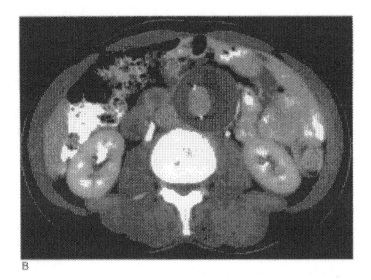

Figure 1. Continued.

limb design, very poor radial force, and essentially uncovered distal stent are probably responsible for this unusual finding. This area does not seem to represent a significant problem for fully supported modular systems, where good apposition can be expected in the iliac vessels, and if not, an extension is readily applied.

Spontaneous resolution also occurs frequently with endoleaks related to branch flow with the majority resolving spontaneously by 6 months. Type II endoleaks seem to persist longer with an unsupported graft such as the Ancure system, as compared to other grafts. Despite this higher initial incidence and subsequent persistence of endoleaks with the Ancure system, there seems to be a significantly higher rate of resorption of the thrombus and shrinkage of the aneurysmal sac as compared to fully supported stent-grafts.

We looked at the rate of aneurysmal sac shrinkage in 70 patients with AAAs that underwent endoluminal treatment with a bifurcated graft between October 1996 and February 1999 at the University of Pittsburgh. The Ancure endograft was used in 43 patients and the Excluder graft in 27 patients. Endoleak rates were 28% with the Ancure system and 18% with the Excluder device. AAA sac regression of >0.5 cm was considered significant and was noted with the Ancure graft in 45% of patients at 6 months and 67% of patients at one year. In comparison a significant regression in sac size was seen with the Excluder graft in only 11% of patients at 6 months and 19% of patients at one year. Our results are corroborated from the literature by several series (22,24).

The differential behavior of the AAA sac with various grafts solely among patients with endoleaks is more difficult to demonstrate from our small numbers. However, it is our clear impression that sacs with endoleak and an Ancure graft seem to shrink frequently while patients with endoleaks and other grafts do not. A reduction in the size of the aneurysm sac implies a reduced amount of tension within the aneurysm sac, but may also be simply related to a different rate of resorption of the clot from the AAA. This rate of resorption may be linked to the rigidity of the endograft associated with stent support or lack thereof among different graft designs. Since an enlargement of the AAA size is a potential prognostic sign leading to intervention, it is clear that differences in the behavior of endoleaks among grafts is of therapeutic importance. Although these early observations should undergo further documentation, they do point to the importance of differentiating similar types of endoleaks based on the endograft in question.

Of note also is that early endoleaks do not seem to influence sac collapse among patients treated with the Ancure endograft. Follow-up of AAA size over time in patients with an endoleak that sealed spontaneously was similar to those who never had an endoleak. At 24-month follow up, 80% of patients with an endoleak that sealed and 76% of patients with no endoleak had shown a significant reduction in size of at least 5 mm by CT scan.

V. TREATMENT OF ENDOLEAKS

Interventions aimed at treating endoleaks have been recommended very early because of the increased risk of rupture if observed for a considerable period of time (13,14,21). The significant rate of spontaneous closure with no intervening complications in our patients appears to justify a policy of observing these endoleaks for a period of 6 months prior to any intervention.

As previously mentioned, proximal attachment system endoleaks are mostly associated with neck angulation in our experience. Twelve such endoleaks were noted with the Ancure system, and 10 of them resolved spontaneously in our patients. Of 2 that required later intervention, one was actually associated with a distal type I endoleak. Distal type I endoleaks with the bifurcated Ancure system occur in the setting of ectatic or tortuous iliac arteries that are somewhat larger than the limbs. An effective seal with the Ancure endograft in this setting is unlikely in the absence of radial apposition to the native vessels provided by stents in the limbs. These leaks tend to be persistent. This decreased apposition provides an unusual access to the AAA sac for treatment not provided by fully supported modular stent-grafts.

Patients with persistent endoleaks undergo angiography and attempted coiling. In our initial series there were a total of 10 such endoleaks, 7 of which required intervention. One patient was treated with an extension endograft because the presence of a Wallstent across the distal anchoring mechanism prevented easy access to the aneurysm sac. The remaining 6 patients with persistent type I distal endoleaks underwent angiography and coiling through the previously mentioned approach. There was only one patient with a persistent type II endoleak, and this too was successfully coiled through an SMA approach. Our subsequent experience remains unchanged. The technique used in coiling these endoleaks has been previously described (23). Briefly, the AAA cavity is accessed around the limb of the Ancure graft and coils deposited in the outflow vessels from the sac. Large coils are next packed in the sac down to the attachment frame. A follow-up CT is obtained at 6–8 weeks, and if a residual endoleak is detected, the procedure is repeated. One patient required three treatment sessions before complete obliteration of the endoleak, attesting to the need for persistence with the technique.

Coiling of the source, outflow, and cavity of the endoleak was successful in all cases in achieving a radiographic seal of the endoleak based on both angiography and CT scanning (Fig. 2). Following successful coiling, all patients showed a decrease in AAA size on follow-up CT scans from 6 to 30 months after obliteration of the leak. The persistent endoleaks associated with the Ancure endograft seem to be particularly well suited for this coiling technique. The body of the graft is unsupported and most persistent endoleaks occur around the iliac limbs with this graft, allowing for relatively easy access to the aneurysm cavity. Coiling through an access around limbs, however, may not be well suited in fully supported modular grafts. The exoskeleton may hamper attempts to access the cavity around the graft and other options may have to considered. Direct translumbar sac puncture and stent graft extensions are modalities that have been used in this setting. The different approaches to treatment highlights another difference of endoleaks among different endografts.

The clinical significance of endoleaks has not been clearly defined. Shrinkage of the aneurysmal sac has been documented in some patients with an endoleak by imaging studies, while others have an expanding AAA with no demonstrable endoleak. The term "endotension" was coined to more accurately describe the clinical scenario of AAA enlargement and the risk of rupture. As yet there is no reliable means of measuring endotension, leaving us with endoleaks or AAA size change as the only indirect measure of treatment success or failure and the potential risk of rupture. Hence, we believe that all persistent endoleaks should be treated, unless the AAA is shrinking and there is a compelling reason, such as an unstable medical state, to do otherwise.

By adopting a policy of 6 months of observation of endoleaks and subsequent coiling of persistent perigraft flow, we have been successful in excluding the aortic aneurysm sac in nearly all patients at 1-year follow-up.

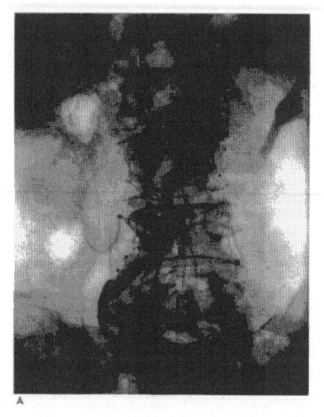

A

Figure 2. (A) Arteriogram demonstrating a type I endoleak originating from the anterolateral aspect of the right distal attachment site of an Ancure endograft. (B) After effective coiling there is no further evidence of endoleak.

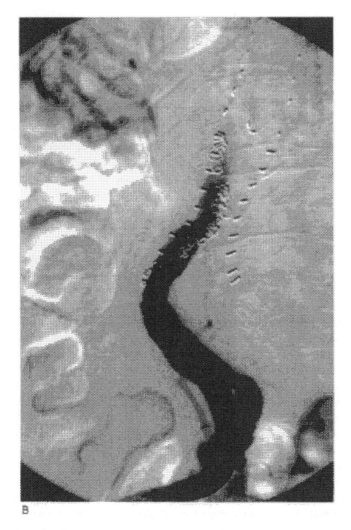

B

Figure 2. Continued.

VI. SUMMARY

Endoleaks remain the Achilles' heel of endovascular exclusion of the AAA
sac from circulation. There is an accumulating body of evidence to suggest
that the origin and behavior of endografts is graft specific, and that proper

management of these endoleaks needs to be tailored to the particular graft system. Certain types of endoleaks are associated with particular devices and are related to the attachment system, modular joint interface, or fabric of the device. Others may be related to the adaptation of endoluminal devices to the change in aortic morphology that occurs over time following endograft placement.

Our experience with two systems seems to indicate a higher initial incidence of endoleaks with the Ancure system as compared to the Excluder. Despite the higher incidence and persistence of endoleaks with the unsupported Ancure system, there appears to be a higher rate of resorption of thrombus and shrinkage of the aneurysmal sac as compared to the fully supported Excluder graft. The site of origin of the endoleak may be of some predictive value when it comes to prognosis. Proximal attachment endoleaks, unless a result of poor technical deployment, are usually associated with an angulated neck, and these leaks appear to spontaneously resolve in just about all cases with the Ancure system. Hence we feel comfortable observing a proximal type I endoleak noted at the time of graft deployment with the Ancure system. This approach differs significantly from the proximal endoleaks noted with fully supported grafts, as these endoleaks are generally treated when they are discovered.

The unsupported nature of the Ancure endograft seems to result in a higher incidence of distal attachment system endoleaks that remain persistent. This same body design, however, also makes access to aneurysm cavity relatively simple, allowing for the use of coiling as a treatment modality. In our hands coil embolization of the aneurysm sac and outflow vessels has been very effective in sealing persistent endoleaks with the Ancure endograft. It has also been very reassuring to observe a subsequent decrease in the aneurysm sac size with the Ancure system. Branch flow endoleaks also appear to resolve spontaneously in the majority of cases.

Established treatment protocols are essential for centers engaging in this treatment modality for AAA. A 6-month period of careful observation appears to be justified since the majority of endoleaks spontaneously resolve within this period without any adverse long-term sequelae. Beyond this period we recommend pursuing an aggressive treatment regimen to obliterate the source of the endoleak and prevent potential rupture of the AAA. A period of further close observation and follow-up may be justified in patients with a shrinking aneurysmal sac or a deteriorating medical condition.

Finally, if an endoleak persists despite these treatment options, the conventional open repair procedure can always be relied upon. The drawback of endoleaks associated with endovascular repair of AAA highlights the need for continued long-term follow-up. The continued study of these endoleaks and their behavior with various endograft systems will hopefully lead to the development of graft-specific treatment protocols.

REFERENCES

1. Moore WE, Kashyap VS, Vescera CL, et al. Abdominal aortic aneurysm: a six-year comparison of endovascular vs transabdominal repair. Ann Surg 1999; 230:20–30.
2. Buth J, Leheij RJF. on behalf of the EUROSTAR Collaborators. Early complications and endoleaks after endovascular abdominal aortic aneurysm repair: report of a multicenter study. J Vasc Surg 2000; 31:134–146.
3. Zarins CK, White PA, Hudgson KJ, Schwarten D, Fogarty TJ. for the AneuRx Clinical Investigators. Endoleak as a predictor of outcome following endovascular aneurysm repair. AneuRx Multicenter Clinical Trial. J Vasc Surg 2000; 32:90–107.
4. Makaroun M, Zajko A, Orons P, et al. The experience of an academic medical center with endovascular treatment of abdominal aortic aneurysms. Am J Surg 1998; 176:198–202.
5. Riepe G, Heilberger P, Unscheid T, Chakfe N, Raitherl D, Stelter W, et al. Frame dislocation of body middle rings in endovascular stent tube grafts. Eur J Endovasc Surg 1999; 17:28–34.
6. Bohm T, Soldner J, Rott A, Kaiser WA. Perigraft leak of an aortic stent graft due to material fatigue. Am J Roentgenol 1999; 172:1355–1357.
7. Krohg-Sorensen K, Brekke M, Drolsum A, Kvernebo K. Periprosthetic leak and rupture after endovascular repair of abdominal aortic aneurysm: the significance of device design for long-term results. J Vasc Surg 1999; 29:1152–1158.
8. Makaroun M, Zajko A, Sugimoto H, et al. Fate of endoleaks after endoluminal repair of abdominal aortic aneurysms with the EVT device. Eur J Vas Endovasc Surg 1999; 18:185–190.
9. Baum RA, Carpenter JP, Cope C, Golden MA, Velacquez O, Neschis DG, Mitchell ME, Barker CF, Farman RM. Aneurysm sac pressure measurements after endovascular repair of abdominal aortic aneurysms. J Vasc Surg 2001; 33:32–41.
10. Ahn SS, Rutherford RB, Johnston KW, May J, Veith FJ, Baker JD, et al. Reporting standards for infrarenal endovascular abdominal aortic aneurysm repair. Ad Hoc Committee for Standardized Repoting Practices in Vascualr Surgery of the Society for Vascular Surgery/International Society for Cardiovascular Surgery. J Vasc Surg 1997; 25:405–410.
11. Chuter TAM, Risber B, Hopkinson BR, Wendt G, Scott RAP, Walker PJ, et al. Clinical experience with a bifurcated endovascular graft for abdominal aortic aneurysm repair. J Vasc Surg 1996; 24:655–666.

12. White GH, May J, Waugh RC, Chaufour X, Yu W. Type III and IV endoleak: toward a complete definition of blood flow in the sac after endoluminal AAA repair. J Endovasc Surg 1998; 5:305–309.

13. White GH, Yu W, May J. "Endoleak": a proposed new terminology to describe incomplete aneurysm exclusion by an endoluminal graft. J Endovasc Surg 1996; 3:124–125.

14. Wain RA, Marin ML, Ohki T, et al. Endoleaks after endovascular graft treatment of aortic aneurysms: Classification, risk factors and outcome. J Vasc Surg 1998; 27:69–80.

15. Resch T, Ivancev K, Lindh M, et al. Persistent collateral perfusion of abdominal aortic aneurysm after endovascular repair does not lead to progressive change in aneurysm diameter. J Vasc Surg 1998; 28:242–249.

16. May J, White GH, Yu W, et al. Endovascular grafting for abdominal aortic aneurysm: changing incidence and indication for conversion to open operation. Cardiovas Surg 1998; 6:194–197.

17. May J, White G, Yu W, et al. A prospective study of anatomic-pathological changes in Abdominal Aortic Aneurysms following endoluminal repair: Is the aneurysmal process reversed? Eur J Vasc Endovas Surg 1996; 12:11–17.

18. Torsello G, Klenk E, Kasprzak B, Umscheid T. Rupture of abdominal aortic aneurysm previously treated by endovascular stentgraft. J Vasc Surg 1998; 28:184–187.

19. Zarins CK, White RA, Fogarty T. Aneurysm rupture after endovascular repair using the AneuRx stent graft. J Vasc Surg 2000; 31:960–970.

20. Franco TJ, Zajko A, Federle M, Makaroun M. Endovascular repair of abdominal aortic aneurysms with the Ancure endograft: CT follow-up of perigraft flow and aneurysm size at 6 month. JVIR 2000; 11:429–435.

21. Moore WS, Rutheford RB. Transfemoral endovascular repair of abdominal aortic aneurysm: results of the North American EVT phase I trial. J Vasc Surg 1996; 23:543–553.

22. Matsumura JS, Pearce WH, McCarthy WJ. Reduction in aortic aneurysm size: early results after endovascular graft placement. J Vasc Surg 1997; 25:113–123.

23. Amesur N, Zajko A, Makaroun M. Embolotherapy of persistent endoleaks following endovascular repair of abdominal aortic aneurysm with the ancure endovascular technologies endograft. J Vasc Surg 1999; 10:1175–1182.

24. Broeders IA, Blankensteijn JD, Gvakharia A, May J, Bell PR, Swedenborg J, Collin J, Eikelboom BC. The efficacy of transfemoral endovascular aneurysm management: a study of size changes of the abdominal aorta during mid-term follow-up. Eur J Vasc Endovasc Surg 1997; 14:84–90.

17

Diagnosis and Treatment of Intraoperative Endoleaks: When Is the Operation Really Over?

Ronald M. Fairman and Omaida C. Velazquez
University of Pennsylvania School of Medicine and University of Pennsylvania Medical Center, Philadelphia, Pennsylvania, U.S.A.

Richard A. Baum
Brigham & Women's Hospital and Harvard Medical School, Boston, Massachusetts, U.S.A.

Although there remains an element of uncertainty and at times overt skepticism regarding the current results of aortic endografting, for the elderly, physiologically disadvantaged patient with a large abdominal aortic aneurysm, the technology has created previously nonexistent options for treatment. The importance of patient selection predicated on meticulous and sophisticated anatomical assessment cannot be overemphasized. The aortic endografting devices have also created a host of new challenges and in some cases major obstacles for practicing vascular surgeons. Even for those individuals experienced in performing endovascular interventions, aortic endografting mandates a learning curve that is often protracted and tedious given the first-generation nature of the two FDA-approved devices. Although the manufacturers of the Ancure (Guidant/Endovascular Technologies, Menlo Park, CA) and AneuRx (Medtronic, Santa Rosa, CA) stent grafts have committed themselves to physician training, all too often appropriate patient selection, meticulous endograft design, and successful deployment of these devices does not result in prompt exclusion of the aneurysm sac. The focus of this chapter is on the diagnosis and treatment of intraoperative endoleaks and, in particular, the approaches and techniques that we have evolved during our first 300 cases performed at the University of Pennsylvania.

The question raised in the title of this chapter, "When is the operation really over?" refers to the situation where the stent graft has been deployed to everyone's satisfaction and yet the completion arteriogram reveals an endoleak. Although these patients are still therapeutically heparinized with activated clotting times of greater than 250 seconds, it is incorrect to automatically assume that the endoleak is merely due to fabric porosity or "blush" (type IV) and that it will resolve with reversal of anticoagulation (Fig. 1).

All intraoperative endoleaks require precise definition and appropriate intervention before the patient leaves the operating room. Often times, diagnosing the precise source of an endoleak is conceptually a more difficult exercise than the adjunctive procedures used to subsequently treat it. Our

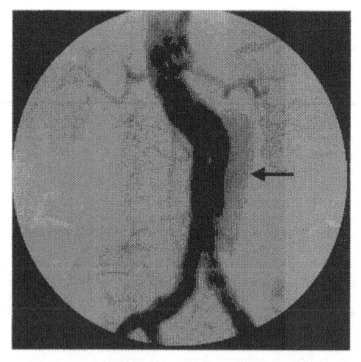

Figure 1. Type IV endoleak.

standard completion arteriogram includes a power injector study in an anterior-posterior projection with a 5 F pigtail catheter positioned just above the proximal attachment site at the level of the renal arteries. Magnification is helpful, but it is important to visualize the entire endograft including all attachment sites during the completion study. Typically the power injector is set up to deliver 20 cc of contrast per second for a total volume of 40 cc. Delay imaging is very important in order to assess collateral lumbar and ilio-lumbar artery flow. When an endoleak is apparent, the first feature to assess is the rate of aneurysm sac filling. Endoleaks that rapidly fill the sac are suggestive of a fixation problem such as a proximal or distal attachment attachment site endoleak (type I), or a junctional issue (type III) (Figs. 2 and 3). Alternatively, delayed, gradual filling of the sac on the completion run is suggestive of a type II endoleak (Fig. 4).

The second feature to focus on is the timing and directionality of lumbar and ilio-lumbar collateral flow in relation to the aneurysm sac. In the presence of a type I or type III endoleak, the sac will fill first and then lumbar arteries

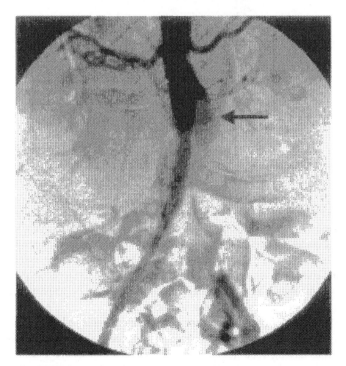

Figure 2.   Proximal attachment site (type I) endoleak.

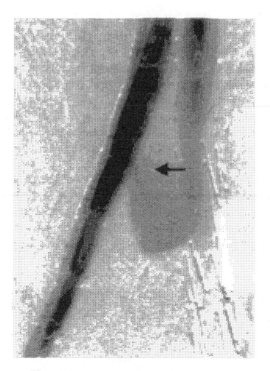

Figure 3. Junctional (type III) endoleak.

will slowly fill as contrast within the sac dissipates. A type II endoleak will first produce filling of lumbar collaterals and subsequent filling of the sac. It is important to play back the digital arteriography image repeatedly and to define the direction of flow in the lumbar and ilio-lumbar arteries. By definition, type II endoleaks are characterized by retrograde flow in collateral lumbar arteries with subsequent delayed filling of the sac. An endoleak that rapidly fills the aneurysm sac and later produces antegrade flow in lumbars is further evidence of a fixation issue (type I or III) that needs further attention. It is essential to analyze and manipulate the completion arteriogram as a dynamic sequence of images, and at times it is particularly helpful diagnostically to play back the images in slow motion, one frame at a time.

If the completion arteriogram demonstrates delayed filling of the aneurysm sac via retrograde flow in lumbar collaterals, the operation is then complete, thus having documented a type II endoleak and secure fixation at the attachment sites and junctions. We do not presently advocate intervention for

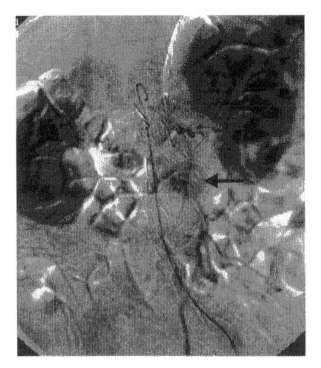

Figure 4.   Type II inferior mesenteric artery endoleak.

type II endoleaks identified on the completion arteriogram. It has been our experience that this finding is not predictive of persistent endoleak at 30 days.

Alternatively, if the sac fills promptly at the same time that the stent graft is filling with contrast, it is likely that an attachment or junctional problem exists. Findings particularly diagnostic of a proximal attachment site endoleak include brisk filling of the sac as the stent graft fills with contrast, prior to contrast reaching the distal attachment sites. A simple diagnostic maneuver is to pull the pigtail catheter down below the proximal attachment site and into the trunk or body of the stent graft and repeat the arteriogram. If the endoleak was due to poor fixation at the proximal attachment site, it will no longer be evident. A persistent brisk endoleak with the pigtail positioned below the proximal attachment site may signal a junction problem (if the stent graft is modular) or poor fixation at one of the distal attachment sites. Alternatively, Figure 5 demonstrates delayed filling of the sac through iliolumbar collaterals (type II) when the pigtail has been pulled down into the right graft limb.

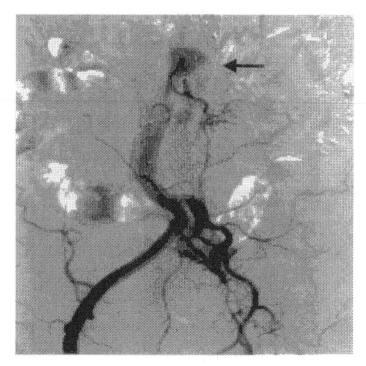

Figure 5. Type II iliolumbar collateral endoleak.

The distal attachment sites may be adequately evaluated by performing a retrograde digital arteriogram using 20 cc of contrast through sheaths placed in both femoral arteries. If the respective distal attachment site is insecure, contrast will be seen to promptly outline the attachment site and fill the sac during the retrograde injection. At times, magnification and oblique projections can be particularly helpful. Once proximal and distal attachment sites have been assessed and found to be secure, all modular stent grafts should have the graft-to-graft junctions imaged in the setting of a persistent endoleak. This is accomplished by changing over to a long radiopaque-tipped sheath and performing a retrograde arteriogram with the tip positioned at the site of the junction. A jet of contrast filling the sac implies that the graft-to-graft junction is unstable.

A summation of this strategy is presented in Table 1. Using this protocol, we have consistently identified the etiology and significance of

Table 1. Diagnostic Features of Intraoperative Endoleaks

Type I
1. Brisk filling of the aneurysm sac as contrast fills the stent graft with the pigtail positioned above the proximal attachment site.
2. Contrast appears in the sac before it is seen filling lumbar and iliolumabar collaterals.
3. Direction of blood flow in lumbar collaterals is antegrade from the sac.
4. If a brisk endoleak disappears when the pigtail is pulled down below the proximal attachment site into the body of the stent graft, the etiology is type I localized to the proximal attachment site.
5. Performing retrograde femoral digital arteriograms through bilateral femoral sheaths best assesses the distal attachment sites.

Type II
1. Delayed filling of the aneurysm sac as contrast washes out of the stent graft with pigtail positioned above the proximal attachment site.
2. Lumbar and iliolumbar collaterals fill first with contrast before the sac is seen to slowly fill with contrast.
3. Blood flow in lumbar collaterals is retrograde into the sac.

Type III
1. Brisk filling of the sac with delayed antegrade washout through lumbar collaterals.
2. Repeat arteriogram with pigtail positioned below the proximal attachment site and within the body of the stent graft still produces brisk endoleak.
3. Performing repeat retrograde digital arteriogram using long radiopaque-tipped femoral sheath positioned at graft-to-graft junction best demonstrates jet of contrast filling the sac.

Type IV
1. Delayed generalized "blush" of contrast through graft fabric with faint antegrade filling of lumbar collaterals.
2. A viable consideration only after first stepwise excluding types I, II, and III endoleak.

intraoperative endoleaks. It is important to stress that a delayed "blush" attributable to fabric porosity and systemic anticoagulation (type IV) is always a diagnosis of exclusion. It should only be considered after stepwise assessment of the attachment sites, junctions, and lumbar collateral flow.

The adjunctive procedures and options available to successfully treat an intraoperative endoleak are dependent upon a number of factors. Typically, the AneuRx modular stent grafts come with a "toolbox" of proximal and distal covered extensions but lack balloons. The extensions allow for fine-tuning fixation at the attachment sites, although an AneuRx proximal covered extension can only be deployed if there exists at least 1 cm distance from the lowest renal artery to the top of the bifurcated main body of the stent graft. Failure to adhere to this strict guideline will trap the septum of the flow divider, resulting in compromised flow to the contralateral limb. The Ancure unibody system comes with a compliant balloon built into the delivery/deployment system, but there are no proximal or distal covered extensions. Although standard teaching dictates that these compliant balloons are safely inflated to 2-atmosphere pressure, we believe this may be a dangerous routine practice. Alternatively, we inflate only to achieve balloon profile. Recognizing these inherent design characteristics of the two FDA-approved stent grafts, we have developed the following strategy for treating intraoperative endoleaks. A summary of these adjunctive interventions is provided in Table 2.

Intraoperative proximal attachment site endoleaks develop under a variety of circumstances, including sizing errors, complicated aortic neck anatomy (Fig. 6), and deployment-related mishaps resulting in distal migration

Table 2. Adjunctive Procedures to Treat Intraoperative Endoleaks

Completion arteriogram	Interventions
Type I endoleak at proximal attachment site	
Accurate proximal graft deployment	Balloon angioplasty (sized to aortic neck)
Migrated proximal graft	
AneuRx	Proximal covered extension
Ancure	Graft within a graft
Type II endoleak at distal attachment site	
Accurate distal graft deployment	Balloon angioplasty (sized to common iliac artery)
Inaccurate distal graft deployment	
AneuRx	Distal covered extension ("bell-bottom")
Ancure	Retroperitoneal suture repair
Type III endoleak	
Proximal AneuRx limb at top of gate	Balloon angioplasty (sized to graft limb)
Migrated AneuRx limb, unstable junction	Covered extension

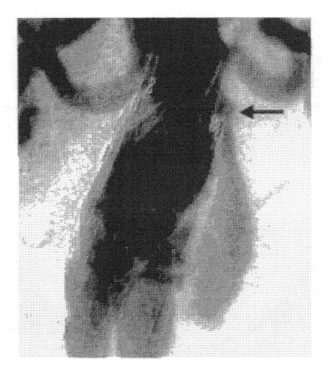

Figure 6. Complicated aortic neck.

(Fig. 7). If the stent graft is in fact well positioned immediately below the lowest renal artery, we will approach these endoleaks by performing a balloon angioplasty at the proximal attachment site. With the recent availability of commercially produced large angioplasty balloons, this has become a simple undertaking (Fig. 8). The balloon should be sized to the diameter of the aortic neck, not the diameter of the stent graft design. Ballooning the neck should be done very tentatively given the potential for aortic neck rupture. Although the Ancure delivery system has a built-in compliant balloon as described above, we typically do not reintroduce the original delivery system after the completion arteriogram, and instead resort to a noncompliant large angioplasty balloon. The placement of an adjunctive short, rigid, balloon-expandable uncovered stent to increase the radial force and help secure better fixation proximally may be another option, but the data on this type of intervention are currently anecdotal.

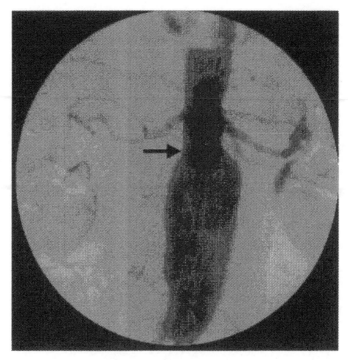

Figure 7. Migrated stent graft.

Alternatively, if the stent graft has migrated downward during deployment producing poor fixation at the top, further intervention is determined by the unibody or modular nature of the stent graft. This can be addressed with a proximal covered extension if one is dealing with an AneuRx modular design. It again needs to be emphasized that at least 1 cm distance must exist between the lowest renal artery and the top of the stent graft to avoid trapping the septum of the flow divider and compromising flow to the contralateral limb. If the stent graft design is an Ancure and the proximal attachment site has migrated during deployment resulting in a type I endoleak, immediate options are somewhat limited. This does not occur commonly. We have found that the proximal hooks deploy accurately, and migration can be prevented by promptly pulling down the balloon across the proximal attachment site and inflating it to profile. The graft is most vulnerable to migration during the time interval between deployment of the proximal hooks and balloon inflation. We have no experience utilizing AneuRx proximal

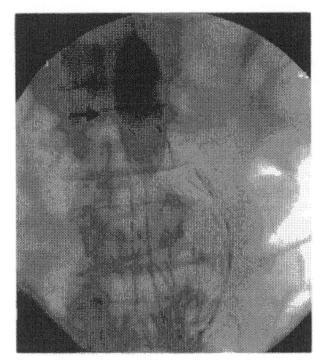

Figure 8.   Balloon angioplasty of proximal attachment site.

aortic cuffs to address Ancure proximal fixation problems, although we are familiar with anecdotal reports. Another potential option to deal with this phenomenon is the "graft within a graft" approach, thereby implanting another Ancure bifurcated graft to achieve more proximal fixation and coverage in the aortic neck.

When the source of the type I endoleak is the distal attachment site, it is most commonly due to graft sizing design error involving anatomical assessment of the common iliac arteries. Our first bifurcated aortic endograft developed a distal ipsilateral attachment site endoleak because we landed too proximally within a dilated common iliac artery that was not appreciated preoperatively. The decision tree for distal attachment site interventions is generally the same as described above for the proximal attachment site. The adjunctive options are the same. If the attachment site is well positioned within the common iliac artery and the graft limb is appropriately sized, performing a balloon angioplasty will often seal the leak. Once again, the angioplasty balloon should be sized to the diameter of the common iliac artery, not the graft limb. In general, we believe one should avoid ballooning across the distal attachment site, as we have experienced two iliac artery ruptures early in our series before we recognized this potential. When one needs to move the attachment site more distally in the common iliac artery to achieve fixation during an AneuRx deployment, one places a distal covered extension. If the leak is due to a sizing error, one may choose to create a "bell-bottom" effect by oversizing the distal extension. Meticulous preoperative anatomical assessment and patient selection are essential when placing the unibody Ancure device given the lack of distal covered extensions. In general, however, we have accepted the philosophy that it is not mandatory for the seal to occur at the distal hooks so long as it does occur somewhere along the course of the common iliac artery. We have on occasion supported Ancure limbs with flexible uncovered self-expanding stents to increase the radial force and improve distal fixation. Alternatively, a retroperitoneal exposure, excising the distal attachment hooks and converting to a sutured anastomosis, may be indicated. We have no experience using AneuRx distal covered extensions to manage Ancure distal attachment issues.

When a type III intraoperative endoleak occurs at the AneuRx contralateral short limb junction, intervention is determined by where the contralateral limb resides within the junction gate. If the proximal end of the contralateral limb rests high up within the gate, then balloon angioplasty alone will seal the junction. Since the graft-to-graft junction typically resides up in the aneurysm sac, the balloon is sized to the diameter of the graft limb. If magnified views reveal that the contralateral limb has dropped down low in the gate during deployment, an appropriately sized self-expanding covered extension limb will be required with the proximal end deployed at the top of the junction gate.

In summary, intraoperative endoleaks require precise definition and appropriate intervention when they are detected on the completion arteriogram. The diagnostic and interventional strategies we have described above have consistently permitted characterization and successful treatment of these endoleaks.

18

Clipping of Inferior Mesenteric and Lumbar Arteries via Retroperitoneal Laparo-Endoscopic Approach as a Treatment of Persistent Endoleak

Willem Wisselink, Miguel A. Cuesta, Abraham Rijbroek, and Jan A. Rauwerda
Vrije University and Vrije University Medical Center, Amsterdam, The Netherlands

I. INTRODUCTION

As type I endoleaks are uniformly considered a reason for urgent reintervention, type II endoleaks generally are being observed since spontaneous thrombosis frequently occurs (1–5). In the case of persistence of the endoleak beyond 6 months with failure of the aneurysm to shrink or increase of aneurysm diameter, however, therapeutic intervention may be indicated (6–8). Catheter embolization of patent lumbar of inferior mesenteric arteries, either alongside the limbs of the graft or via superior mesenteric or hypogastric arteries, had proven to be a valuable treatment option (9). However, this method may not be technically feasible in all cases due to tortuosity of the collateral circulation or multiplicity of patent connections to the aneurysm sac. Efficacy of direct injection of thrombogenic material into the aneurysm sac is debated since pressure in the aneurysm may remain unaltered (10,11). Recently, we reported a laparoscopic approach for treatment of a patient in whom treatment of persistent type II endoleak was deemed necessary and catheter embolization unlikely to succeed (12). In this chapter we describe in detail our surgical technique as well as the early clinical results of clipping of lumbar and inferior mesenteric arteries via a laparo-endoscopic, retroperitoneal approach as a minimally invasive surgical treatment option for persistent type II endoleak.

II. PATIENTS AND METHODS

Between August 1999 and November 2000, 5 patients (all men) presented with persistent type II endoleak more than 6 months (13 ± 5 months) following endovascular repair (EVR). The mean aneurysm diameter (5.7 ± 0.5 cm) had remained unchanged since the operation in four patients and slightly increased (2 mm in 18 months) in one. Aneurysm volume in this patient had increased from 125 cc directly postoperatively to 132 cc at 18 months. Angiography revealed three ($n = 1$), four ($n = 3$), or six ($n = 1$) patent lumbar arteries, whereas the inferior mesenteric artery was patent in four of five patents. One patient had developed vague abdominal and back pain, the remaining were a symptomatic. Significant comorbidities were insulin-dependent diabetes mellitus ($n = 1$) and intermittent atrial fibrillation with chronic anticoagulant use ($n = 1$). Prosthetic devices used were AneuRx (Medtronic/AVE Corporation, Santa Rosa, CA) ($n = 4$) and Endovascular Technologies (EVT, Guidant Corporation, Menlo Park, CA) ($n = 1$). In one patient, catheter embolization had been attempted both via hypogastric collaterals and alongside the iliac limbs, without success. Following approval from the institutional human ethics committee, all patients were treated with retroperitoneal endoscopic ligation of lumbar and inferior mesenteric arteries.

A. Operative Technique

Under general anesthesia, the patient is placed on a "bean bag" in a 60 degrees right lateral decubitus position. The region between the left costal margin and the iliac crest is maximally extended by flexing the operating table. The surgeon and assistant are standing on the left side of the patient facing the monitor on the opposite side. The tip of the twelfth rib is palpated and an incision of 2 cm length made just anteriorly. With the help of a clamp and index finger, a small space is created in two directions, posteriorly by mobilizing the lower pole of the kidney and anteriorly towards the umbilicus. A dissecting balloon (Origin Medsystems, Menlo Park, CA) is introduced and the balloon insufflated in order to enlarge the created retroperitoneal space, thereby mobilizing the lower pole of the kidney anteriorly. As the camera is inserted into the balloon, the left ureter is coming into view. In the latest three cases, an additional 10 mm trocar has been inserted intraabdominally via the umbilicus allowing dissection of the retroperitoneum under direct vision. This technique is also helpful in case small perforations of the peritoneum occur since air can be drained out of the abdominal cavity, allowing full deployment of the retroperitoneal space. The dissecting balloon is replaced by a 10 mm trocar and the retroperitoneum insufflated with carbon dioxide up to a pressure of 14 mmHg. A 0-degree videoendoscope is introduced through the cannula and two additional trocars of 10 mm diameter each are placed, one close to the iliac crest in the posterior axillary line, the other near the costal margin, in the anterior axillary line in order to create a wide working space and avoid "instrument crowding" (Fig. 1). After identification of the psoas muscle, the left ureter is being mobilized anteriorly and the infrarenal aorta exposed from the left renal artery to the iliac bifurcation. Measurement of intra-aneurysm pressure was attempted by means of insertion of a laparoscopic needle attached to a pressure monitor. Following dissection of the posterior aspect of the aneurysm, the left-sided lumbar arteries are

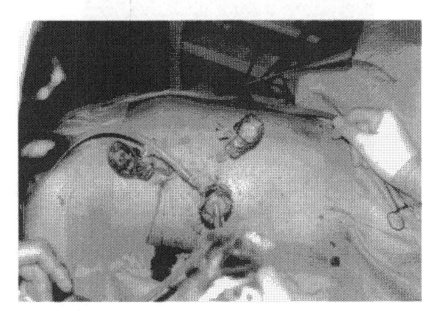

Figure 1.   Patient position on the operating table with three trocars in retroperitoneal space. The head is to the right.

identified, ligated, and divided using medium-size titanium clips (Endoscopic Rotating Multiple Clip Applier®, Ethicon Endo-Surgery, Cincinnati, OH) (Fig. 2). Subsequently, the aneurysm can be slightly tilted to facilitate identification of the right lumbar arteries, which are clipped and left undivided (Fig. 3). If indicated, the anterior surface of the aneurysm is exposed and the inferior mesenteric artery identified and clipped (Fig. 4).

B. Postoperative Management

Spiral computed tomography–angiography (CTA) was performed on the first postoperative day, at 3, 6, and 12 months, and semi-annually thereafter (Fig. 5).

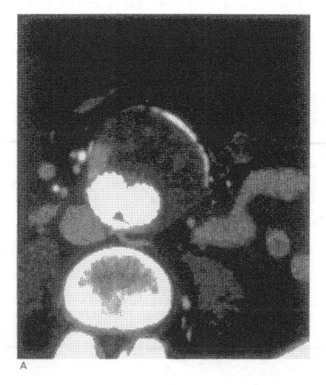

A

Figure 2. (A) CT-angiography: endoleak present at 8 months follow-up. (B) Angiography, same period: multiple patent lumbar arteries.

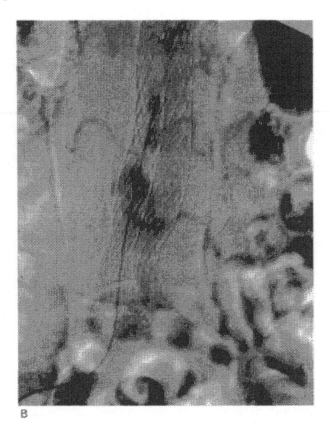

B

Figure 2.   Continued.

III. RESULTS

There were no deaths and no complications. Mean operative time was 128 minutes (100–160); all patients were removed from mechanical ventilation immediately postoperatively without the need for admission to an intensive are unit. Regular diet was resumed 1 ($n = 4$) or 2 ($n = 1$) days after the operation and all patients left the hospital within 4 days after the operation. Postoperative spiral CT scan ($n = 5$) revealed, in one patient, pair of unclipped, patent lumbar arteries. Following immediate reoperation via the same approach with clipping of the remaining pair of lumbar arteries just at the aortic bifurcation, complete thrombosis of the aneurysm sac was

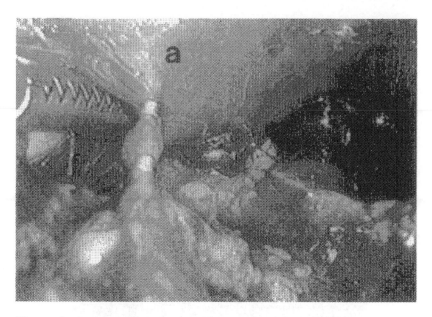

Figure 3.   Laparo-endoscopic view of the AAA with clipped lumbar artery. a, aneurysm.

radiographically confirmed. Another patient continued to have an endoleak in spite of absence of patent branch arteries. By subsequent angiography, contrast appeared to originate at the proximal attachment site, thus constituting a type I endoleak. Thirteen months following laparoscopic clipping, the appearance of the endoleak, as well as the aneurysm diameter and volume, have remained unaltered by CT scanning. The option of conversion to open repair has been considered, however, the patient to date has refused. In the remaining patients ($n = 3$) complete exclusion of the aneurysm sac was demonstrated at the first postoperative scan. With a mean follow-up of 11 ± 7 months, 4 of 5 patients have remained free from endoleak, whereas aneurysm diameter has remained unchanged in 3 and decreased (7 mm in 8 months) in one.

IV. DISCUSSION

The high incidence of endoleaks remains one of the most vexing dilemmas associated with endovascular repair of abdominal aortic aneurysm (AAA) (1–

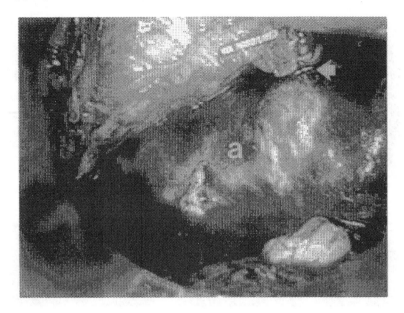

Figure 4.   The inferior mesenteric artery has been dissected free and clipped (arrow). a, aneurysm. (Figure graciously provided by J. C. Parodi, MD.)

5). The natural history of this complication is insufficiently known, and indications for therapy are therefore not well established. Type I endoleaks, as most authors agree, require immediate therapy and, if endoluminal maneuvers do not suffice, conversion to open repair. Type II endoleaks, on the other hand, initially believed to be associated with a lower residual pressure in the aneurysm sac (endotension), may spontaneously thrombose and, therefore, be observed initially. Disconcerting, however, is the study by Baum et al. who percutaneously inserted catheters in to the aneurysm sac in patients with type II endoleak and found systemic pressures without exception. Furthermore, aneurysm rupture following EVR is being reported with increasing frequency even in patients without a demonstrable endoleak (4,10,11). Transcatheter embolization of patent lumbar or inferior mesenteric arteries, either alongside the limbs of the graft or via superior mesenteric of hypogastric arteries, has been well described (9). However, with multiple patent lumbar arteries present, as was seen in our small series, this technique has failed us in one patient and was not attempted in the others. Following the first operation in this series, CTA continued to reveal contrast in the aneurysm sac as well as one pair of patent lumber arteries just proximal to the iliac bifurcation. At

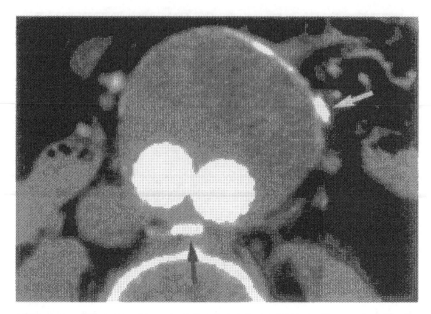

Figure 5. CT angiography: absence of endoleak, titanium clips on lumbar, and mesenteric arteries (arrows).

immediate reoperation, dissection was relatively simple and the remaining pair of patent lumbar arteries could easily be identified and clipped. This experience has made it clear that to ensure that all lumbar arteries are addressed, the entire posterior surface of the aneurysm needs to be dissected free, allowing a clear, uninterrupted view of the inferior vena cava in the background. In principle, only those lumbar arteries that contribute to the endoleak need to be ligated. In future cases, where accurate identification of a small number of patent branch arteries might allow less extensive dissection, concurrent fluoroscopy and angiography on the operative table may be used towards this end. The role of endopressure as a means to judge completeness of lumbar ligation remains unclear. In our series, we used a small, short laparoscopic needle and did not attempt selective cannulation of the liquid portion of the aneurysm, party for technical reasons but also for of fear for bleeding in absence of hemostatic tissues embedding the dissected aneurysm wall. Continuous pressure registration revealed a straight line, without a pulse wave or other fluctuations in the three cases it was attempted, probably due to the fact that the needle tip was embedded in thrombus. Therefore, safe and simple techniques to measure intrasac pressure, also in thrombus, are sorely needed. In the one patient who continued to have an endoleak, a type I component probably had been present prior to the laparoscopic procedure but not recognized as such due to the multiple patent branch arteries. It is not inconceivable that the situation has actually been made worse by occluding the outflow of the aneurysm sac in the presence of a type I endoleak.

In this chapter, a novel retroperitoneal endoscopic approach to persistence of a type II endoleak following endovascular AAA repair has been demonstrated. This procedure may be a less invasive alternative to open repair in those patients in whom transcatheter embolization has been unsuccessful or is likely to fail. Obviously, however, to validate this approach, long-term follow-up of a large series is required.

ACKNOWLEDGMENTS

The authors gratefully acknowledge Jan D. Blankensteijn, MD, and Juan C. Parodi, MD, for contributing their follow-up data.

REFERENCES

1. White GH, May J, Waugh RC, Chaufour X, Yu W. Type III and IV endoleak: toward a complete definition of blood flow in the sac after endoluminal AAA repair. J Endovasc Surg 1998; 5(4):305–309.
2. Laheij RJ, Buth J, Harris PL, Moll FL, Stelter WJ, Verhoeven EL. Need for secondary interventions after endovascular repair of abdominal aortic aneurysms. Intermediate-term follow-up results of a European collaborative registry (EUROSTAR). Br J Surg 2000; 87(12):1666–1673.
3. Schurink GW, Aarts NJ, van Bockel JH. Endoleak after stent-graft treatment of abdominal aortic aneurysm: a meta-analysis of clinical studies. Br J Surg 1999; 86(5):581–587.
4. Cuypers P, Buth J, Harris PL, Gevers E, Lahey R. Realistic expectations for patients with stent-graft treatment of abdominal aortic aneurysms. Results of European multicentre registry. Eur J Vasc Endovasc Surg 1999; 17(6):507–516.
5. Schurink GW, Aarts NJ, van Baalen JM, Chuter TA, Schultze Kool LJ, van Bocke JH. Late endoleak after endovascular therapy for abdominal aortic aneurysm. Eur J Vasc Endovasc Surg 1999; 17(5):448–450.
6. Gorich J, Rilinger N, Sokiranski R, Kramer S, Schutz A, Sunder-Plassmann L. Pamler R. Embolization of type II endoleaks fed by the inferior mesenteric artery: using the superior mesenteric artery approach. J Endovasc Ther 2000; 7(4):297–301.

7. Baum RA, Carpenter JP, Tuite CM, Velazquez OC, Soulen MC, Barker CF, Golden MA, Pyeron AM, Fairman RM. Diagnosis and treatment of inferior mesenteric arterial endoleaks after endovascular repair of abdominal aortic aneurysms. Radiology 2000; 215(2):409–413.

8. Karch LA, Henretta JP, Hodgson KJ, Mattos MA, Ramsey DE, McLafferty RB, Sumner DS. Algorithm for the diagnosis and treatment of endoleaks. Am J Surg 1999; 178(3):225–231.

9. Amesur NB, Zajko AB, Orons PD, Makaroun MS. Embolotherapy of persistent endoleaks after endovascular repair of abdominal aortic aneurysm with the ancure-endovascular technologies endograft system. J Vasc Interv Radiol 1999; 10(9):1175–1188.

10. Schurink GW, Aarts NJ, Van Baalen JM, Kool LJ, Van Bockel JH. Experimental study of the influence of endoleak size on pressure in the aneurysm sac and the consequences of thrombosis. Br J Surg 2000; 87(1):71–78.

11. Marty B, Sanchez LA, Ohki T, Wain RA, Faries PL, Cynamon J, Marin ML, Veith FJ. Endoleak after endovascular graft repair of experimental aortic aneurysm: does coil embolization with angiographic "seal" lower intraaneurysmal pressure? J Vasc Surg 1998; 27(3):454–462.

12. Wisselink W, Cuesta MA, Berends FJ, Berg van den FG, Rauwerda JA. Retroperitoneal endoscopic ligation of lumbar and inferior mesenteric arteries as a treatment of persistent endoleak following endoluminal aortic aneurysm repair. J Vasc Surg 2000; 31:1240–1244.

13. Baum RA, Carpenter JP, Cope C, Golden MA, Velazquez OC, Neschis DG, Mitchell ME, Barker CF, Fairman RM. Aneurysm sac pressure measurements after endovascular repair of abdominal aortic aneurysms. J Vasc Surg 2001; 33(1):32–41.

14. Torsello GB, Klenk Kasprzak B, Umscheid T. Rupture of abdominal aortic aneurysm previously treated by endovascular stentgraft. J Vasc Surg 1998; 28(1):184–187.

19

The Inferior Mesenteric Artery as a Principal Source of Backflow Endoleaks: Incidence and Management

Omaida C. Velazquez and Ronald M. Fairman
University of Pennsylvania School of Medicine and University of Pennsylvania Medical Center, Philadelphia, Pennsylvania, U.S.A.

Richard A. Baum
Brigham & Women's Hospital and Harvard Medical School, Boston, Massachusetts, U.S.A.

I. INTRODUCTION

Since first introduced, the endovascular repair of infrarenal aortic aneurysms has been gaining increased acceptance as favorable early-outcome reports increase in numbers and feasibility reports proliferate, expanding the anatomical indications for this approach (7,16,19–21,24,40). Despite the strong enthusiasm for this new method, the consistent findings of high postprocedure endoleak rates (up to 21%) appears to represent a real and poorly understood problem (3–6,9,11,13,14,17,25,29,33–37,39). Data presented from the EVT (Endovascular Technologies) and Medtronic trails at an FDA panel indicated up to 48% endoleak rates on early CT scan follow-up. While great concern has been expressed over persistent anchoring site (type I) endoleaks (particularly proximal endoleaks), little is known about the significance of type II endoleaks (related to the inferior mesenteric artery, lumbars, and other collateral vessels) (1). Data from the EUROSTAR registry on 1554 patients from 1994 to 1999 documented a 16% rate of endoleaks detected at the completion of the procedure and a 9% rate of endoleaks one month after the procedure. A significant percentage of endoleaks (related to anchoring sites or collateral vessels) appear to spontaneously disappear after variable periods of follow-up, whereas new endoleaks, not previously observed, may appear on a delayed fashion (3,8,18). Therefore, the time interval that defines a persistent endoleak that triggers concern varies widely among investigating centers. Even after the endoleak thromboses and is no longer detectable on computed tomography (CT) scan, it is unknown whether this occurrence eliminates transmitted pressure through the unexcluded thrombus to the aneurysm sac. If there remains transmitted systemic pressure to unexcluded aneurismal aorta, one might anticipate that, analogous to an unrepaired thrombosed aneurysm, the risk of rupture would remain. Some patients with persistent endoleaks have been reported to experience progressive aneurysm dilatation and fatal rupture (38). Even more perplexing are the reported cases where an endoleak is not detectable by conventional radiographic imaging techniques, but the aneurysm sac continues to expand and/or the patient incurs aneurysm rupture (12). Thrombus within the aneurysm sac may transmit both mean and pulse pressure to the wall of the aneurysm, and therefore thrombus alone may not be protective against aneurysm expansion and rupture. For example, aortic aneurysms thrombosed by ligating the iliac arteries may still go on to rupture. Schurink et al. (25–30) measured the pressure within the aneurysmal thrombus, at its thickest point, in nine patients undergoing open repair of infrarenal aortic aneurysms. They noted that both mean and pulse pressures within the thrombus were similar to systemic pressure measurements. However, in a pig experimental model where 16 saccular aneurysms were connected to the aorta by branches of varying lengths and diameters (simulating different size collateral-endoleaks), the thrombosed or partially thrombosed aneurysm sacs were not systemically pressurized. In this experimental mode, an open branch "endoleak" of any size was capable of producing pulsatile systemic pressure within the aneurysm sac, independent of the size of the "endoleak." Pulsatile systemic pressure within these experimental aneurysms sacs were successfully obliterated be either spontaneous thromboses of the "endoleak" or Gelfoam or Histoacryl glue induced thromboses the "endoleak" but not the sac. However, the mean aneurysm pressure after thrombosis was significantly increased as the diameter of the thrombosed "endoleak" was increased, again suggesting that thrombus can transmit pressure if the diameter of the conduit (collateral branch) is sufficiently wide. If the "endoleak" remained open, the sac remained pressurized, regardless of whether or not the aneurysm sac was thrombosed.

Since the risk of aneurysm rupture in different types of endoleak is unknown, investigators at different centers have arbitrarily opted to follow patients with different types of endoleaks for time intervals ranging from days to months to more than one-year periods. It has been assumed by many currently investigating this new minimally invasive procedure that only persistent proximal endoleaks carry the ongoing risk of aneurysm rupture. However, an increasing number of published and unpublished anecdotal reports indicate that patients may go on to rupture their abdominal aortic aneurysm after what has been thought to be successful endovascular aneurysm exclusion, and even with documented aneurysm size reduction. Not all reports are clearly connected to just proximal anchoring site endoleaks. For mainly this reason, careful long-term follow-up has been advocated by many, as we learn more about the effectiveness and durability of this new method of aneurysm repair. Recently, an in vitro study suggested that even a small collateral vessel (0.410 mm) could maintain systemic pressure within an excluded aneurysm sac model (29).

Flow from the inferior mesenteric artery (IMA) in a retrograde fashion through superior mesenteric artery (SMA) collaterals, or in an antegrade fashion through lumbar inflow, is responsible for a significant number of type II endoleaks and may result in transmitted systemic pressures into the aneurysm sac (2–4). In our early studies we focused on IMA-related type II endoleaks. Our goal was to begin to characterize the incidence and clinical significance of IMA-related type II endoleaks (2,3). We aimed to answer specific questions of relevance to both doctors and patients:

1. To what extent does preoperative IMA patency, on radiographic imaging, represent a predictor of postoperative IMA endoleaks after endovascular repair of infrarenal aortic aneurysm?
2. Can an IMA endoleak transmit systemic pressure to the aneurysm sac?
3. Can an IMA endoleak be safely and successfully obliterated via the endovascular approach after primary stent-grafting?
4. Is there reason to attempt preoperative IMA embolization, when the vessel is seen to be patent by preoperative imaging modalities?

II. PREOPERATIVE DETERMINATION OF IMA PATENCY

IMA patency was defined as visualization of this vessel in communication with the aneurysm as seen by preoperative imaging, which included a contrast

CT angiography, conventional contrast arteriogram, and, in selected patients (those with chronic renal insufficiently), magnetic resonance angiography. Diagnostic magnetic resonance imaging/magnetic resonance angiography (MRI/MRA) replaced CT scan/contrast arteriogram in five patients because of an elevated creatinine. All radiographic studies were retrieved and independently rereviewed in a blinded fashion by an expert radiologist (3,4).

III. ASSESSMENT FOR ENDOLEAKS

In the operating room, after implanting the device, the proximal and distal anchoring sites were individually studied by antegrade and retrograde arteriograms to identify anchoring site endoleaks. If such an anchoring site problem was identified, additional ballooning, stenting, or addition of covered extensions was performed until the operating surgeon was thoroughly satisfied that an anchoring site endoleak was completely ruled out. At this point, a power injection completion antegrade arteriogram, with delayed imaging, was performed. An endoleak was defined as any visualized contrast (including faint blush) filling the aneurysm sac outside of the stent-graft. Postoperative CT scans (150 cc of iodinated contrast material at 4 cc/s using spiral 3-mm cuts with a pitch of 2) were performed prior to discharge and at one month of follow-up. Views obtained from these CT scans included pre-contrast injection, dynamic, and delayed contrast images, which were reviewed for the presence or absence of endoleaks, using both the printed films and a three-dimensional work station. Some patients were studied postoperatively by ultrasound, which can be useful in documenting the presence or absence of an endoleak. However, we observed early in our experience that in many patients the postoperative ultrasound study was suboptimal or inconclusive.

IV. DETERMINATION OF ENDOLEAK ETIOLOGY

Further diagnostic/therapeutic arteriograms were performed in patients with 30-day persistent endoleaks, aimed at clearly identifying the source of the endoleak. In our experience, CT scan and ultrasound modalities were insufficient for accurately determining the type of endoleak present. Since most centers now agree that a type I endoleak may essentially represent an untreated abdominal aortic aneurysm (AAA), it is the authors' philosophy that in the setting of an endoleak that has persisted for 30 days, one needs to rule out the presence of a type I endoleak. With this rationale, selective and supra-selective arteriograms were utilized to accurately diagnose the source of all endoleaks noted to persist beyond 30 days after endovascular AAA repair. When technically feasible, this modality was also utilized therapeutically to obliterate endoleaks. These arteriograms were undertaken as a methodical and objective evaluation. First, an antegrade arteriogram via proximally placed 5 French pigtail catheter, specifically looking for proximal anchoring site endoleaks, was performed. Anterior-posterior and lateral intra-arterial digital subtraction aortograms were performed with the pigtail positioned at the proximal stent-graft anchoring site, filming at 3 frames per second and continued until contrast was completely washed out of the arterial and venous systems. Similar arteriograms were repeated with the pigtail moved to the graft-to-graft attachment sites. Retrograde arteriograms via distal femoral sheaths looking for distal anchoring site endoleaks were then performed. After excluding anchoring site or graft-to-graft endoleaks, selective *SMA and hypogastric artery* angiograms, looking for endoleaks related to collateral circulation (IMA or lumbars, respectively), were performed. At this time, a microcatheter was advanced into the aneurysm sac (when technically feasible) and pressure measurements were obtained. Also, at this time selective embolization of the collateral vessel causing the endoleak was performed when feasible, as described below.

V. TREATMENT OF TYPE II ENDOLEAKS AND MEASUREMENT OF ANEURYSM SAC PRESSURES

In investigating and treating IMA-related endoleaks, a 4 or 5 French catheter was placed at the proximal neck of the SMA and an external coaxial tracker (3 French, 150 cm microcatheter (Fast Tracker, Boston Scientific, Natick, MA) was used to cannulate the middle colic artery. The Tracker catheter was advanced through the middle colic and IMA into the aneurysm sac. After a hand-injected digital run was performed to confirm the origin of the endoleak, intrasac pressure measurements were made and compared to systemic arterial pressure, measured noninvasively at the level of the brachial arteries. The high resistance of the catheter system and the anatomical tortuosity of the collateral vessels en route to the IMA in most cases precluded measurement of systolic, diastolic, and pulse pressures. In those patients, mean pressure was, therefore, recorded for comparison with mean systemic pressure.

The microcatheter was then withdrawn to the proximal portion of the IMA, where microcoils were deployed until radiographic evidence of stasis of blood flow was obtained. Subsequent SMA arteriograms were performed to confirm elimination of the endoleak. Postembolization CT scans were also performed to examine the aneurysm sac and confirm the complete obliteration of the endoleak.

In our initial experience with 76 consecutive cases, there were a total of 13 (17%) 30-day persistent endoleaks on postoperative CT scans at one month of follow-up (4). Only 5 of these were noted in the operating room on completion of power injection arteriogram. The remaining 8 of these were not detected by the operating room completion arteriogram. Conversely, 17 patients with evidence of endoleak on completion arteriogram in the operating room subsequently had no evidence of endoleak on follow-up CT scans.

With the use of CT scan plus standard and selective angiography, 11 of 13 (85%) endoleaks persisting at thirty days were confirmed to be related to collateral circulation form the IMA into the aneurysm sac. Lumbars and/or branches of the hypogastric arteries were often identified as sources of outflow by injecting contrast directly into the aneurysm sac through the same catheter used to measure aneurysm sac pressure. There was one proximal and one distal anchoring site endoleak (2.6% overall, 15% of all endoleaks). During the course of this study, all patients with persistent flow through the aneurysm sac were noted to have patent lumbar arteries serving as egress vessels (including the two patients with type I endoleaks), but antegrade flow into the aneurysm sac from a lumbar artery source was not seen in this series of patients, despite thorough evaluation that included selective hypogastric artery arteriography.

Anchoring site endoleaks were repaired with covered stent-graft extensions as secondary endovascular procedures.

In a study of IMA patency by preoperative angiogram and preoperative CT scan in patients with and without postoperative IMA endoleaks, 50% of patients with an IMA-associated endoleak had a preoperative patent IMA by angiography. Only 27% of those patients without an endoleak had an angiographically patent IMA. This difference did not reach statistical significance. Ninety percent of patients with an IMA-related endoleak had a preoperative patent IMA by CT scan versus only 48% of those without an endoleak. This difference was statistically significant. Twenty-four percent of patients with a patent IMA by preoperative CT scan versus only 3% of those without a patent IMA (by preoperative CT scan) suffered from IMA-related type II endoleaks that persisted at 30-days after stent-graft repair of their AAA ($p < 0.05$).

To determine whether one can predict postoperative IMA-related endoleaks based on IMA patency by preoperative imaging, the sensitivity, specificity, predictive value, and accuracy of the imaging modalities were calculated assuming that a 30-day persistent IMA endoleak was the gold standard measure of clinically relevant IMA patency. Sensitivity was best for CT scan alone at 90%. Specificity and accuracy were best for concurring readings on CT scan and angiogram. Negative predictive value was high with all single and combination imaging modalities (highest for CT scan alone at 97%). Positive predictive value and accuracy were uniformly low (4).

In 8 of the 11 patients with an IMA-related 30-day persistent endoleak, the aneurysm sac pressure was measured using a catheter technique. Six of these patients had systemic pressures within the aneurysm sac. In the remaining three patients, the measurement of sac pressure was not technically feasible, related to vessel caliber and tortuosity resulting in inability to advance the microcatheter.

When the IMA is identified as the source of type II endoleaks, it can be successfully embolized in most patients via an SMA approach (5,14,17,32). Selective embolization of the IMA was possible with subsequent obliteration of the IMA-related endoleaks in 9 to 11 patients. In the other two patients, one endoleak thrombosed spontaneously at one-month of follow up and one patient expired from severe preexisting hepatic dysfunction. All patients with subselective embolization of the IMA angiographic resolution of the endoleaks and negative one-month follow-up CT scans. In this series, all patients surviving currently are free of endoleaks, with 13 of 76 (17%) patients having required secondary endovascular procedures aimed at obliterating 30-day persistent endoleaks.

VI. DISCUSSION

A significantly higher proportion of patients whose preoperative CT scan demonstrates a patent IMA suffer from postoperative IMA-related endoleaks compared to those whose preoperative CT scan *did not show* a patent IMA [9/38 (24%) vs. 1/32 (3%); $p < 0.05$] (4). Similarly, a significantly higher proportion of patients with an IMA-related endoleak had a patent IMA visualized by preoperative CT scan compared to patients without an endoleak [9/10 (90%) vs. 29/60 (48%); $p < 0.035$]. The preoperative identification of a patent IMA on arteriogram did not have a similar predictive value. The preoperative identification of a patent IMA on CT scan, therefore, was associated with a statistically and clinically significantly higher proportion of patients with postprocedural type II endoleak (which included inflow from the IMA and outflow through patent lumbar arteries).

In a clinical sense, however, a useful significant predictor of postoperative type II endoleak would be able to discriminate which of the patients with a patent IMA would be most likely to suffer from an IMA-related type II endoleak (i.e., would be a clinical test with high positive predictive value and high accuracy). An analysis of the preoperative imaging studies alone and in combination demonstrates that the positive predictive value and accuracy are not sufficiently high to discriminate clinically between patients in such groups. That is, in patients where the preoperative imaging indicates a patent IMA, the majority *will not* go on to suffer from an IMA-related endoleak. For these reasons, preoperative interventions (e.g., embolization of the IMA) based on the preoperative imaging studies are not advocated by the authors, since this would result in many unnecessary interventional procedures. This recommendation is further strengthened by our success with the postoperative endovascular obliteration of IMA endoleaks via selective embolization in those patients with persistent endoleaks.

Although it might be considered intuitive or "self-evident" that patients with nonpatent IMA should not develop IMA-related endoleaks, it is reassuring that the data bear out this expected finding while demonstrating the constrains of the overall incidence of false positives and false negatives and the global sensitivity, specificity, and accuracy of the preoperative imaging studies as they demonstrate the status of the IMA. Because radiographic imaging data depend on technical aspects of the performance of the study as well as the subjective interpretation of the radiologist, we believe that the statistical analysis performed bears significant relevance to the question of whether a clinician can trust such data for the purposes of patient information and/or predictions as to the potential trouble with IMA-related endoleak. While it is true that less than a quarter of patients who had a radiographically patent IMA went on to develop an IMA-related endoleak, it is also true that a statistically and clinically significant higher ratio of patients with a patent IMA (radiographically) went on to develop an IMA endoleak when compared to the group of patients that had a radiographically nonpatent IMA.

We have also identified in our series that intraoperative endoleaks visualized on completion arteriogram are not necessarily predictive of postoperative persistent endoleaks visualized on follow-up CT scans. Since the standard nonselective aortogram does not appear to be the best method for detecting endoleaks, and since many collateral branches may thrombose spontaneously between the completion arteriogram and the first postoperative CT scan, we were not surprised to find little correlation between the endoleaks seen in the operating room completion arteriogram and those seen on postoperative CT scans.

With the measurements of aneurysm sac pressure in patients who had IMA-related endoleaks, we have established the feasibility of this technique and demonstrated that a significant number of patients with an IMA endoleak continue to have systemic pressure within the aneurysm sac (2,4). The presence of the microcatheter within the IMA may actually lead to alterations in the detected pressure within the aneurysm sac (by virtue of the microcatheter partially occluding flow within the patent IMA). The authors believe that this may in fact account for the lower pressure recorded in the two patients and the overall decreased pulse pressure noted within the aneurysm sac. However, this is only a speculation, and the data available are insufficient to determine with certainty what might be the etiology or clinical significance of the measured pressures. Further studies are clearly warranted on this subject. Moreover, in view of the fact that intrasac pressures were not measured in any patient in whom there was not a postoperative endoleak, one cannot be absolutely certain that the patent IMA is the only cause of the high intrasac pressure. As will be discussed below, it is unlikely that the high intrasac pressures were maintained by patent lumbar arteries in these studied patients given the angiographic evidence. Alternatively, it might be possible that the pressure may be actually transmitted through the fabric wall into the aneurysm sac.

In our series we noted an overall 30-day persistent endoleak rate of 17%, which is within the range of what others have reported (3,5,9,25–29), but we have a preponderance of type II endoleaks, all of which have been IMA-related endoleaks (IMA identified as inflow, lumbar arteries visualized and likely to represent outflow, as discussed below). We would have expected a higher rate of anchoring site endoleaks, given that 46% of patients enrolled had extreme unfavorable anatomy for endovascular repair, but this was not seen possibly due to our preference for suprarenal fixation and the preponderant use of modular devices which allow for easy intraoperative repair of detected anchoring-site leaks. This distribution of endoleak etiology has not been frequently noted by other investigators. One may postulate that such a difference reflects a sampling variability related to a different set of patients with a differing range of aneurysm anatomical features, differences in the types of endoprosthesis utilized, or differences in fixation choice (the majority of our patients were repaired with suprarenal bare-spring fixation). However, it is more likely that our methodical and extensive study designs aimed at clearly identifying the exact endoleak inflow source accounts for our findings. This rigorous, objective approach that we have pursued for the identification of endoleak etiology has not been previously undertaken. Most prior reports have not utilized postoperative selective angiography in the pursuit of endoleak etiology. Most authors have relied on postoperative CT scans and ultrasound in the evaluation of postoperative endoleaks (3,18–23).

In many patients, the anatomical variability of where the collateral vessels enter/exit the aneurysm sac precludes an exact localization of the endoleak inflow source when only using CT or ultrasound imaging, even with the use of dynamic spiral CT angiography with three-dimensional reconstruction, although in one patient we were able to clearly demonstrate the endoleak source using this latter modality. Standard antegrade anterior-posterior and lateral aortography was also limited in many cases, in terms of clearly localizing the source of endoleaks. One case (a proximal endoleak) was diagnosed by this latter modality without need for further selective images. However, most cases required selective angiography to clearly identify the endoleak inflow source. In some patients with CT scan evidence of an endoleak, no obvious contrast blush was noted by standard aortography. In these cases, selective arteriograms revealed the small but definite contrast extravasation into the aneurysm sac. In all cases a source of egress from the sac was noted through small lumbar or hypogastric artery branches.

In our series, lumbars, branches from the hypogastrics, or accessory renals were not seen to fill the aneurysm sac antegrade as a primary source of a type II endoleak. Since many patients showed these branches to be patent on preoperative angiogram and CT scan, we believe these were small enough to have thrombosed after stent-grafting or, when patent, did not show antegrade flow into the aneurysm sac but rather appeared to serve as egress vessels. Similarly, many patients with a patent IMA on preoperative imaging did not show an IMA-related endoleak, presumably as a result of thromboses of this vessel after stent-grafting.

In all cases where the IMA was noted to produce an antegrade contrast blush in the aneurysm sac, lumbar branches were identified as egress vessels on delay filming. As a matter of traditional radiographic convention, we have attributed the cause of the endoleak to the source of inflow (in our series the IMA). Other groups have reported a higher rate of lumbar artery-related type II endoleaks. Thus, one may question whether some of the endoleaks observed in our series have inflow through the lumbar arteries. However, the selective hypogastric arteriograms fail to indicate antegrade flow from lumbar branches in aneurysm sac. The type II endoleaks noted were identified only on selective SMA/IMA arteriogram. It would be unlikely that contrast dye injected under pressure through a catheter located in the IMA would diffuse through the aneurysm sac and then flow against systemic pressure, into the lumbar arteries. This contrast would then follow retrograde, against systemic pressure, into the patent lumbars and drain through the venous system only if the lumbars represented a low pressure system acting as an outflow for the endoleak. The authors feel certain that the collective data obtained from the thorough selective and subselective arteriography was sufficient to precisely identify the nature and source of the endoleak at hand in each individual patient. Therefore, it was concluded that in the series herein reported, the type II endoleaks observed thus far show inflow from the IMA and outflow through the lumbar arteries. To the extent that flow through an endoleak mandates both inflow and outflow (from a high-pressure system to a low-pressure system), the patent lumbar arteries contributed to the endoleak. However, selective embolization of the IMA has resulted in successful obliteration of the endoleak (by angiography and CT scan) in all cases thus far.

While most agree that anchoring site endoleaks represent a failure to successfully repair the aneurysm by the endovascular method, the significance of type II endoleaks remains unknown and there is no consensus for a standard of treatment (3,5,10,13,15,22,23,28,31). Some have reported success with embolization of the feeding collateral vessel responsible for the endoleak, while others have advocated embolization of the aneurysm sac itself. This latter method continues to carry the question of whether systemic pressure can be transmitted through clot to the aneurysm aortic wall. In some cases the option has been to observe without treatment depending on feasibility and success of secondary procedures. In Zarins et al.'s report, 9% of patients continued to have an endoleak at 6 months of follow-up, but no endoleaks were seen on CT scan at 15 months of follow-up (39). They report no aneurysm ruptures during follow-up and evidence of aneurysm size decrease from 6.5 to 5.0 cm in one patient at 1 year of follow-up despite persistence of the endoleak. Other authors have also noted lack of aneurysm growth on short-term follow-up despite persistent endoleaks. However, it is difficult to interpret what this means for an individual patient, since some authors report aneurysm rupture despite successful stent-grafting and in the presence of aneurysm size decreases. Is it possible that to some degree we are rediscovering the natural history of untreated or partially treated abdominal aortic aneurysms?

In our series one patient who had a symptomatic aneurysm (pain and tenderness) continued to have symptoms until a type II endoleak was successfully treated by coil embolization of IMA. Another patient with an endoleak (of unknown etiology) at discharge expired suddenly after collapsing with abdominal pain at home, prior to the one-month follow-up CT scan. This patient had a 7.5 cm aneurysm with minimal thrombus within the sac. With a patent endoleak, the pulse pressure within the experimental aneurysm sac is clearly related to the absence or presence of thrombus within the sac.

Schurink's in vitro model elegantly demonstrated that every endoleak, even a very small one, not visualized by digital subtraction angiography or computed tomographic angiography caused greater than systemic diastolic pressure within the aneurysm sac. Our data have shown that IMA endoleaks can result in systemic pressure within the aneurysm sac. For these reasons we have opted for the approach that the aneurysm is not completely repaired until the patient is endoleak-free. Recognizing that it may take days before all the small collaterals thrombose and knowing that in fact a significant number do thrombose at 30 days of follow-up, we have chosen one month as our follow-up interval prior to elective secondary endovascular procedures aimed at diagnosis and potential treatment. Our primary concern and clinical rationale for the 30-day selective arteriogram for persistent endoleaks was the ability to rule out anchoring site endoleaks. Our premise has been that anchoring site endoleaks may behave as untreated AAA. Thirty days represent an arbitrary interval that lies within what one might consider to be a reasonable waiting time period for elective open repair (to date the standard method of treatment). In a sac without thrombus, the larger the diameter of the branch vessel, the larger the pulse pressure transmitted to the aneurysm sac. However, one might stipulate, based on our experience, that this interval may need to be shortened in patients with symptomatic aneurysms or those with very large aneurysms and little thrombus within the aneurysm sac. Others may contend that this interval is too aggressively short and may choose to follow these patients for longer periods, provided the aneurysm does not progressively expand.

In summary, a significant number of type II endoleaks are caused by a patent IMA. IMA endoleaks can transmit systemic pressure to the aneurysm sac. Selective SMA angiography appears to be the most effective method to identify IMA endoleaks. The preoperative CT scan can be useful in predicting risk of IMA-related endoleaks, but its accuracy and positive predictive value are not sufficiently high to advocate preemptive IMA embolization. Selective coil embolization of the IMA can safely and successfully obliterate persistent IMA endoleaks after aortic stent-grafting. The physiology and clinical significance of endoleaks needs further study.

REFERENCES

1. Ahn SS, Rutherford RB, Johnston KW, May J, Veith FJ, Baker JD, Ernst CB, Moore WS. Reporting standards for infrarenal endovascular abdominal aortic aneurysm repair. Ad Hoc Committee for Standardized Reporting Practices in Vascular Surgery of The Society for Vascular Surgery/International Society for Cardiovascular Surgery. J Vasc Surg 1997; 25(2):405–410.

2. Baum RA, Carpenter JP, Cope C, Golden MA, Velazquez OC, Neschis DG, Mitchell ME, Barker CF, Fairman RM. Aneurysm sac pressure measurements after endovascular repair of abdominal aortic aneurysms. J Vasc Surg 2001; 33(1):32–41.

3. Baum RA, Carpenter JP, Golden MA, Velazquez OC, Clark TW, Stavropoulos SW, Cope C, Fairman RM. Treatment of type 2 endoleaks after endovascular repair of abdominal aortic aneurysms: comparison of transarterial and translumbar techniques. J Vasc Surg 2002; 35(1):23–29.

4. Velazquez OC, Baum RA, Carpenter JP, Golden MA, Cohn M, Pyeron A, Barker CF, Criado FJ, Fairman RF. Relationship between preoperative patency of the inferior mesenteric artery and subsequent occurrence of type II endoleak in patients undergoing endovascular repair of abdominal aortic aneurysms. J Vasc Surg 2000; 32(4):777–788.

5. Baum RA, Carpenter JP, Tuite CM, Velazquez OC, Soulen MC, Barker CF, Golden MA, Pyeron AM, Fairman RM. Diagnosis and treatment of inferior mesenteric arterial endoleaks after endovascular repair of abdominal aortic aneurysms. Radiology 2000; 215(2):409–413.

6. Baum RA, Cope C, Fairman RM, Carpenter JP. Translumbar embolization of type 2 endoleaks after endovascular repair of abdominal aortic aneurysms. J Vasc Interv Radiol 2001; 12(1):111–116.

7. Broeders IA, Blankensteijn JD, Gvakharia A, May J, Bell PR, Swedenborg J, Collin J, Eikelboom BC. The efficacy of transfemoral endovascular aneurysm management: a study on size changes of the abdominal aorta during mid-term follow-up. Eur J Vasc Endovasc Surg 1997; 14(2):84–90.

8. Buth J. Endovascular repair of abdominal aortic aneurysms. Results from the EUROSTAR registry. EUROpean collaborators on Stent-graft Techniques for abdominal aortic Aneurysm Repair. Semin Interv Cardiol 2000; 5(1):29–33.

9. Carpenter JP. Regarding: "The incidence and natural history of type I and II endoleak: A 5-year follow-up assessment with color duplex ultrasound scan". J Vasc Surg 2002; 35(3):595–597.

10. Dias NV, Resch T, Malina M, Lindblad B, Ivancev K. Intraoperative proximal endoleaks during AAA stent-graft repair: evaluation of risk factors and treatment with Palmaz stents. J Endovasc Ther 2001; 8(3):268–273.

11. Fairman RM, Carpenter JP, Baum RA, Larson RA, Golden MA, Barker CF, Mitchell ME, Velazquez OC. Potential impact of therapeutic warfarin treatment on type II endoleaks and sac shrinkage rates on midterm follow-up examination. J Vasc Surg 2002; 35(4):679–685.

12. Fillinger MF. Postoperative imaging after endovascular AAA repair. Semin Vasc Surg 1999; 12(4):327–338.

13. Gilling-Smith GL, Martin J, Sudhindran S, Gould DA, McWilliams RG, Bakran A, Brennan JA, Harris PL. Freedom from endoleak after endovascular aneurysm repair does not equal treatment success. Eur J Vasc Endovasc Surg 2000; 19(4):421–425.

14. Gorich J, Rilinger N, Sokiranski R, Kramer S, Schutz A, Sunder-Plassmann L, Pamler R. Embolization of type II endoleaks fed by the inferior mesenteric artery: using the superior mesenteric artery approach. J Endovasc Ther 2000; 7(4):297–301.

15. Haulon S, Willoteaux S, Koussa M, Gaxotte V, Beregi JP, Warembourg H. Diagnosis and treatment of type II endoleak after stent placement for exclusion of an abdominal aortic aneurysm. Ann Vasc Surg 2001; 15(2):148–154.

16. Henretta JP, Karch LA, Hodgson KJ, Mattos MA, Ramsey DE, MeLafferty R, Sumner DS. Special iliac artery considerations during aneurysm endografting. Am J Surg 1999; 178(3):212–218.

17. LaBerge JM, Sawhney R, Wall SD, Chuter TA, Canto CJ, Wilson MW, Kerlan RK, Gordon RL. Retrograde catheterization of the inferior mesenteric artery to treat endoleaks: anatomic and technical considerations. J Vasc Intervent Radiol 2000; 11(1):55–59.

18. Lundbom J, Hatlinghus S, Wirsching J, Amundsen S, Staxrud LE, GjLlberg T, Hafsahl G, Oskarsson W, Krohg SK, Brekke M, Myhre HO. Endovascular treatment of abdominal aortic aneurysms in Norway: the first 100 patients. Eur J Vasc Endovasc Surg 1999; 18(6):506–509.

19. Marin ML, Hollier LH, Avrahami R, Parsons R. Varying strategies for endovascular repair of abdominal and iliac artery aneurysms. Surg Clin North Am 1998; 78(4):631–645.

20. Marin ML, Parsons RE, Hollier LH, Mitty HA, Ahn J, Temudom T, D'Ayala M, McLaughlin M, Depalo L, Kahn R. Impact of transrenal aortic endograft placement on endovascular graft repair of abdominal aortic aneurysms. J Vasc Surg 1998; 28(4):638–646.

21. Marin ML, Veith FJ. Images in clinical medicine. Transfemoral repair of abdominal aortic aneurysm. N Engl J Med 1994; 331(26):1751.

22. Martin ML, Dolmatch BL, Fry PD, Machan LS. Treatment of type II endoleaks with Onyx. J Vasc Interv Radiol 2001; 12(5):629–632.

23. Mehta M, Ohki T, Veith FJ, Lipsitz EC. All sealed endoleaks are not the same: a treatment strategy based on an ex-vivo analysis. Eur J Vasc Endovasc Surg 2001; 21(6):541–544.

24. Parodi JC, Palmaz JC, Barone HD. Transfemoral intraluminal graft implantation for abdominal aortic aneurysms. Ann Vasc Surg 1991; 5(6):491–499.

25. Schurink GW, Aarts NJ, Malina M, van Bockel JH. Pulsatile wall motion and blood pressure in aneurysms with open and thrombosed endoleaks—comparison of a wall track system and M-mode ultrasound scanning: an in vitro and animal study. J Vasc Surg 2000; 32(4):795–803.

26. Schurink GW, Aarts NJ, van Baalen JM, Chuter TA, Schultze Kool LJ, van Bocke JH. Late endoleak after endovascular therapy for abdominal aortic aneurysm. Eur J Vasc Endovasc Surg 1999; 17(5):448–450.

27. Schurink GW, Aarts NJ, van Baalen JM, Kool LJ, Van Bockel JH. Experimental study of the influence of endoleak size on pressure in the aneurysm sac and the consequences of thrombosis. Br J Surg 2000; 87(1):71–78.

28. Schurink GW, Aarts NJ, van Bockel JH. Endoleak after stent-graft treatment of abdominal aortic aneurysm: a meta-analysis of clinical studies. Br J Surg 1999; 86(5):581–587.

29. Schurink GW, Aarts NJ, Wilde J, van Baalen JM, Chuter TA, Schultze Kool LJ, van Bockel JH. Endoleakage after stent-graft treatment of abdominal aneurysm: implications on pressure and imaging—an in vitro study. J Vasc Surg 1998; 28(2):234–241.

30. Schurink GW, van Baalen JM, Visser MJ, van Bockel JH. Thrombus within an aortic aneurysm does not reduce pressure on the aneurysmal wall. J Vasc Surg 2000; 31(3):501–506.

31. Stelter W, Umscheid T, Ziegler P. Three-year experience with modular stent-graft devices for endovascular AAA treatment. J Endovasc Surg 1997; 4(4):362–369.

32. van Schie G, Sieunarine K, Holt M, Lawrence-Brown M, Hartley D, Goodman MA, Prendergast FJ, Khangure M. Successful embolization of persistent endoleak from a patent inferior mesenteric artery. J Endovasc Surg 1997; 4(3):312–315.

33. Wain RA, Marin ML, Ohki T, Sanchez LA, Lyon RT, Rozenblit A, Suggs WD, Yuan JG, Veith FJ. Endoleaks after endovascular graft treatment of aortic aneurysms: classification, risk factors, and outcome. J Vasc Surg 1998; 27(1):69–80.

34. Walker SR, Halliday K, Yusuf SW, Davidson I, Whitaker SC, Gregson RH, Hopkinson BR. A study on the patency of the inferior mesenteric and lumbar arteries in the incidence of endoleak following endovascular repair of infra-renal aortic aneurysms. Clin Radiol 1998; 53(8):593–595.

35. White GH, May J, Waugh RC, Chaufour X, Yu W. Type III and type IV endoleak: toward a complete definition of blood flow in the sac after endoluminal AAA repair. J Endovasc Surg 1998; 5(4):305–309.

36. White GH, May J, Waugh RC, Yu W. Type I and Type II endoleaks: a more useful classification for reporting results of endoluminal AAA repair [letter] [see comments]. J Endovasc Surg 1998; 5(2):189–191.

37. White GH, Yu W, May J. Endoleak—a proposed new terminology to describe incomplete aneurysm exclusion by an endoluminal graft. J Endovasc Surg 1996; 3(1):124–125.

38. Zarins CK, White RA, Fogarty TJ. Aneurysm rupture after endovascular repair using the AneuRx stent graft. J Vasc Surg 2000; 31(5):960–970.

39. Zarins CK, White RA, Hodgson KJ, Schwarten D, Fogarty TJ. Endoleak as a predictor of outcome after endovascular aneurysm repair: AneuRx multicenter clinical trial. J Vasc Surg 2000; 32(1):90–107.

40. Zarins CK, White RA, Schwarten D, Kinney E, Diethrich EB, Hodgson KJ, Fogarty TJ. AneuRx stent graft versus open surgical repair of abdominal aortic aneurysms: multicenter prospective clinical trial [see comments]. J Vasc Surg 1999; 29(2):292–308.

20

Endoleaks and Endotension: The Malmö Perspective

Timothy Resch
Malmö University Hospital, Malmö, Sweden

Björn Sonesson, Krassi Ivancev, and Martin Malina
Lund University and Malmö University Hospital, Malmö, Sweden

I. ENDOLEAKS

Endoleaks are considered one of the major complications after aortic stent-grafting. The initial classification published by White and coworkers subdivided endoleaks into two major groups (1): graft-related (type I) and non–graft-related (type II). Since then, the endoleak classification has evolved mainly due to the introduction of new stent-graft technology with modulated stent-graft (SG) and thin-walled graft fabric (2). However, the original, simplified classification still gives a solid basis for understanding the impact of endoleaks on stent-graft outcome. The most recent addition of importance to the classification is so-called endotension, which is described in a separate section below.

A. Type I Endoleaks

Initial experience with aortic stent-grafting displayed many type I endoleaks (3). Inadequate patient selection, e.g., short and anatomically difficult aneurysm necks and tortuous iliac arteries, largely caused this. Combined with inferior stent-graft characteristics (e.g., poor proximal and distal fixation, inadequate columnar support, material fatigue and inexperience with stent-graft delivery), this led to a high incidence of type I endoleaks (4).

Refinement of selection criteria and improved operator skills reduced the occurrence of such iatrogenic leaks. However, the new, fully supported, modular stent-grafts have introduced new problems. First, as stent-grafts have become more longitudinally rigid, there is a tendency for the seal between the stent-graft and the proximal neck to become inadequate. If the neck is severely angulated (within itself or between the neck and the aneurysm), the stent-graft will act like a spring and stand at an angle in the neck, causing poor approximation. This phenomenon can be corrected by placing giant balloon-expandable stents such as the Palmaz stent (Cordis/Johnson & Johnson, Warren, NJ) in the proximal portion of the stent-graft (Fig. 1). This stent acts

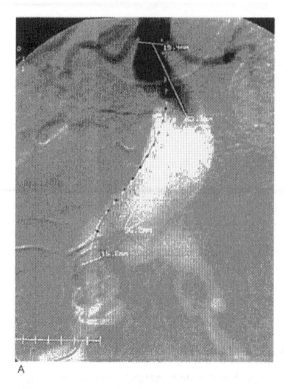

A

Figure 1. (A) Preoperative aortogram demonstrating an angulation between the neck and the aneurysm. (B) Intraoperative aortogram showing malalignment between the stent-graft and the angulated neck, resulting in proximal perigraft endoleak (arrow) in spite of balloon dilatation. (C) Repeated intraoperative aortogram after placement of giant Palmaz stent dilated with 30 mm balloon, no longer showing any perigraft endoleak.

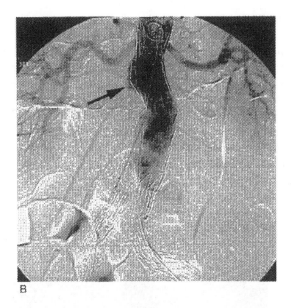

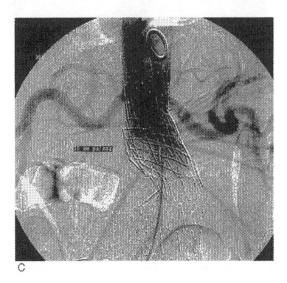

Figure 1. Continued.

as a rigid cylinder that forces the stent-graft to adapt to the aortic wall, thereby obliterating the leak. We have used this technique successfully in several cases. Second, the modular design of stent-grafts allows leaks originating at the modular junctions. If these occur intraoperatively, they can be corrected immediately by ballooning or further SG placement. However, type I leaks can also appear during follow-up as a result of stent-graft migration (5). Mostly, this can be dealt with endovascularly or with external laparascopic banding of the aneurysm (6). Alternatively, a bifurcated endograft can be converted into a monoiliac SG (Fig. 2). When all else fails, open conversion may remain the only treatment option.

Type I endoleaks must be treated vigorously at an early stage to prevent the risk of delayed rupture (7). Anecdotal reports of spontaneous sealing of type I endoleaks must be viewed with great caution. The use of high-quality imaging equipment during stent-graft delivery can aid early diagnosis and

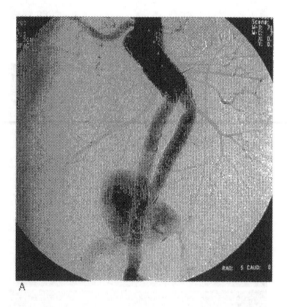

A

Figure 2. (A) Aortogram demonstrating large stent-graft–related endoleak due to separation of stent-graft components. Note also a distal migration of the main body of the stent-graft. (B) Intraoperative aortogram after placement of a uni-iliac stent-graft to the left, resulting in renewed AAA exclusion. (C) Magnified view of intraoperative aortogram, demonstrating the position of the new uni-iliac stentgraft, placed very close to the single kidney renal artery, which has to be stented to preserve patency.

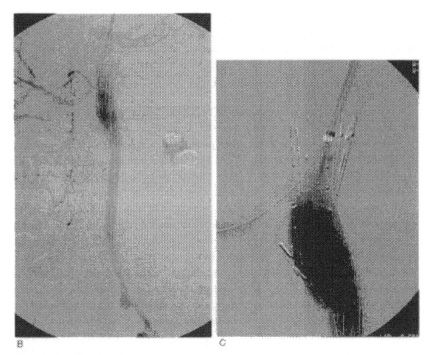

Figure 2. Continued.

usually gives the option of sealing the leak intraoperatively. Even so, follow-up with contrast enhanced spiral computed tomography (CT) 1–3 months after the procedure should be performed to verify a secure stent-graft fit. If a type I leak is then found, it should be further characterized by performing angiography, which also provides a means for endovascular endoleak treatment.

B. Type II Endoleaks

Type II (non–graft-related) endoleaks result from perfusion of the aneurysm sac by collateral vessels such as lumbar arteries or the inferior mesenteric artery. Collateral perfusion is a well-known phenomenon after aneurysm ligation and extra-anatomical bypass. Resnikoff et al. reported a 2% incidence of aneurysm sac perfusion by collaterals in 831 patients treated with this procedure (8). Surgical treatment due to rupture or abdominal pain was required in 41% of these patients. Clinical studies confirm that the incidence of collateral leaks is between 0% and 25% after endovascular exclusion (9). The difference in incidence in these reports is probably a result of differences in imaging. Different techniques (CT, spiral CT, digital subtraction angiography, Duplex scanning) and different protocols for the techniques (slice thickness, contrast volume and concentration, delay) play a major role in identifying these often quite small type II leaks.

It seems as if the presence of type I endoleaks may also have an impact on the incidence of type II endoleaks. The "high-pressure" type I leak serves as the inflow using the ilio-lumbar branches as outflow vessels (10). Subsequently, closure of a type I endoleak may result in thrombosis and disappearance of the type II endoleak. This reasoning also implies that the presence of a type II endoleak suggests that a type I endoleak exists and must be found.

The fate of persistent collateral perfusion is poorly understood. Some aneurysms indeed enlarge during persistent collateral perfusion, but we found that patients with persistent perfusion displayed no significant change in aneurysm diameter during 18-month follow-up. It is noteworthy that, after successful treatment or spontaneous resolution of the perfusions, aneurysms decrease in diameter, suggesting that the perfusion counteracts aneurysm retraction (11). Experimental data imply that a radiographic sealing of a type II leak does not reduce the pressure within the aneurysm sac to the level of a completely excluded aneurysm (12,13). Clinically, we have started measuring intrasac pressure through percutaneous translumbar puncture in patients with type II leaks, and preliminary data indicate that pulsatile pressure transmission is high in patients with enlarging aneurysms (Fig. 3). The increased pulsatile wall motion of the sac found in these patients also supports this (14). Final conclusions from these data and their clinical implications are yet to be drawn as the baseline level of intrasac pressure in completely excluded aneurysms is not fully characterized. Until data are fully analyzed, a cautious attitude is advisable.

Problems associated with type II endoleaks seem to be more an integral part of the technique than those associated with type I leaks (which are often caused by stent-graft or operator failure) are. Better selection might be an option to reduce the number of perfusions. Patients with collateral perfusion have significantly less thrombus in the aneurysm sac preoperatively than patients without perfusion (9). Thrombus placed posteriorly within the sac might be even more protective (15). This suggests either that intra-aneurysmal thrombus acts as a seal to branch vessels or that perhaps the clotting is in some way impaired in patients that develop perfusion leaks. However, a broad overlap between the groups makes preoperative discrimination difficult and exact estimations of thrombus amount and distribution within the entire aneurysm make the measurements unreliable. Others have shown that the

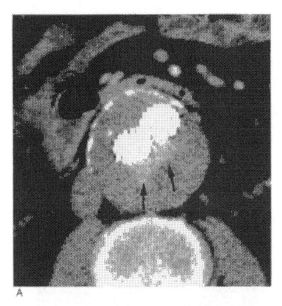

Figure 3.   (A) CT 6 months after Zenith stent-graft AAA repair, showing type II endoleak (arrows). (B) Superselective angiography confirms the iliolumbar perfusion–type II endoleak. Embolization of both outflow and inflow lumbar arteries was successfully performed. (C and D) One year later, repeated CT and selective angiography showed persistent type II endoleak (not shown). Intra-aneurysmal pressure measurement using translumbar approach showed high pressure (mean pressure 66 mmHg to be compared to 99 mmHg systemic pressure). Intra-aneurysmal sac embolization using glue resulted in nonpulsatile tracing and reduction of mean pressure to 14 mmHg, i.e., exclusion pressure.

Continued

preoperative number of patent collateral vessels is a poor predictor of collateral perfusion development (16). Preoperative coil embolization of lumbar arteries seems to have little effect on the development of perfusion endoleaks (17). Other preventive measures to avoid perfusions, such as intraoperative filling of the aneurysm sac with thrombogenic material in patients that have collateral flow intraoperatively, have been proposed and tested with encouraging short-term results (18).

Since preoperative identification of patients likely to develop collateral perfusion is difficult at present and the success of preventive treatment is questionable, the only option is to treat the problem once it appears.

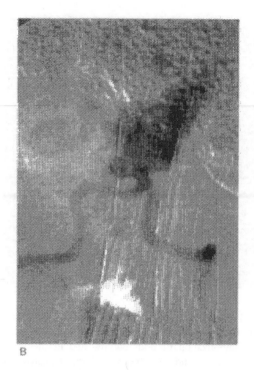

B

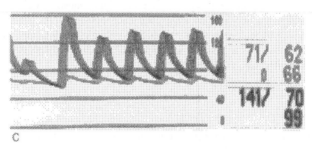

C

Figure 3. Continued.

Transcatheter embolization has been used in some cases, but is not always
successful (Fig. 3). In addition, it exposes patients to an invasive procedure
with the risk of complications. At our institution, one patient suffered transient
paraplegia after such a procedure. Other investigators have tried more
extensive aneurysm packing with coils postoperatively and have found this a

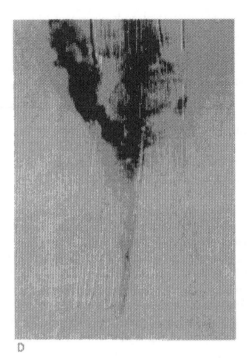

D

Figure 3. Continued.

useful procedure with seemingly few complications (19). Another alternative is translumbar aneurysmal embolization with thrombin or glue (Fig. 3).

In summary, patients that develop type II endoleaks are hard to identify preoperatively and the importance of these leaks for long-term durability of endovascular stent-grafting is unknown. Preliminary experimental and clinical data suggest that they may not have a completely benign course. Continued close observation and evaluation of these patients is required. Methods of identifying patients prone to collateral perfusion and further development of intraoperative abdominal aortic aneurysm (AAA) packing with thrombogenic material might lead to a decrease in the frequency of this complication.

II. ENDOTENSION

Recently, the term "endotension" has been coined to describe an increase in AAA diameter without evidence of endoleak, migration, and/or separation of stent-graft components after stent-graft placement (20). This condition has been ascribed to pressure transmission across thrombus formation between the stent-graft and the arterial wall. In turn, this thrombus prevents demonstration of endoleaks, i.e., accumulation of contrast medium in the aneurysm sac outside the stent-graft. An alternative explanation is that it may represent difficulty in visualizing type II endoleaks, i.e., ilio-lumbar perfusion with currently available imaging modalities (21). In a series of 145 patients successfully treated by endovascular AAA repair, we were able to identify only two patients with aneurysm enlargement fulfilling the criteria of endotension. One patient displayed a thrombosed stent-graft limb in a Vanguard system, caused by stent-graft migration (22). During thrombolytic therapy, a retrograde bleeding with concomitant increase of the aneurysm size occurred. Upon ceasing thrombolytic therapy, the aneurysm again decreased in size. The second patient had a progressive dilatation of the proximal neck with a suprarenal aneurysm formation. After displaying an initial decrease in size of the AAA, the aneurysm subsequently started increasing in size. In both of these patients, a thrombus providing hemostatic seal in the proximal neck appears to transmit continuous pressurization of the aneurysm sac.

Based on these data, we presently believe that aneurysm expansion after SG repair without demonstrable endoleak is caused either by perfusion of the sac or transmission of pressure through thrombosed channels. However, there are anecdotal reports of expanding aneurysms where no such etiology was identified. It is therefore hypothesized that endotension may also be caused by osmotic pressure, transudation through the graft fabric, or a foreign body reaction.

As stated above, it is presently unknown what impact endotension actually has. However, the growth of aneurysms is a real and very disturbing occurrence. The current strategy employed by us is that any aneurysm that begins to enlarge during follow-up must be treated with great caution. A rigorous search for any endoleak must be made and, if found, treated accordingly. If no endoleak is detected, the best treatment option is likely to be open conversion because the risk of aneurysm rupture in the face of continuous aneurysm growth is judged to be high.

REFERENCES

1.   White GH, Yu W, May J, Chaufour X, Stephen MS. Endoleak as a complication of endoluminal grafting of abdominal aortic aneurysms: classification, incidence, diagnosis and management. J Endovasc Surg 1997; 4:152–168.

2. White G, May J, Waugh R, Chaufour X, Yu W. Toward a complete definition of blood flow in the sac after endoluminal AAA repair. J Endovasc Surg 1998; 5:305–309.
3. May J, White G, Yu W, et al. Importance of graft configuration in outcome of endoluminal aortic aneurysm repair: a 5-year analysis by the life table method. Eur J Vasc Endovasc Surg 1998; 15:406–411.
4. Schurink GW, Aarts NJ, van Bockel JH. Endoleak after stent-graft treatment of abdominal aortic aneurysm: a meta-analysis of clinical studies. Br J Surg 1999; 86(5):581–587.
5. Umscheid T, Stelter W. Time-related alterations in shape, position and structure of self-expanding, modular aortic stent-grafts: a 4-year single center follow-up. J Endovasc Surg 1999; 6:17–32.
6. Sonesson B, Montgomery A, Ivancev K, Lindblad B. Fixation of infrarenal aortic stent-grafts using laparascopic banding—an experimental study in pigs. Eur J Vasc Endovasc Surg 2001; 21:40–45.
7. Matsumura J, Moore W. Clinical consequences of periprosthetic leak after endovascular repair of abdominal aortic aneurysm. J Vasc Surg 1998; 27:606–613.
8. Resnikoff M, Darling Rr, Chang BB, et al. Fate of the excluded abdominal aortic aneurysm sac: long-term follow-up of 831 patients. J Vasc Surg 1996; 24:851–855.
9. Resch T, Ivancev K, Lindh M, et al. Persistent collateral perfusion of abdominal aortic aneurysm after endovascular repair does not lead to progressive change in aneurysm diameter. J Vasc Surg 1998; 28:242–249.
10. Broeders I, Blankensteijn J, Eikelbloom B. The role of aortic side branches in the pathogenesis of endoleaks after endovascular aneurysm repair. Eur J Vasc Endovasc Surg 1998; 16:419–426.
11. Malina M, Ivancev K, Chuter T, et al. Changing aneurysmal morphology after endovascular grafting: relation to leakage or persistent perfusion. J Endovasc Surg 1997; 4:23–30.
12. Schurink G, Aarts N, Wilde J, et al. Endoleakage after stent-graft treatment of abdominal aneurysm: implications on pressure and imaging—an in vitro study. J Vasc Surg 1998; 28:234–241.
13. Marty B, Sanchez L, Ohki T, et al. Endoleak after endovascular graft repair of experimental aortic aneurysms: Does coil embolization with angiographic "seal" lower intraaneurysmal pressure? J Vasc Surg 1998; 27:454–462.
14. Malina M, Länne T, Ivancev K, Lindblad B, Brunkwall J. Reduced pulsatile wall motion of abdominal aortic aneurysms after endovascular repair. J Vasc Surg 1998; 27(4):624–631.
15. Armon M, Yusuf S, Whitaker S, Gregson R, Wenham P, Hopkinson B. Thrombus distribution and changes in aneurysm size following endovascular aortic aneurysm repair. Eur J Vasc Endovasc Surg 1998; 16:472–476.
16. Walker S, Halliday K, Yusuf S, et al. A study of the patency of the inferior mesenteric and lumbar arteries in the incidence of endoleak following

endovascular repair of infra-renal aortic aneurysms. Clin Radiol 1998; 53:593–595.

17. Gould D, McWilliams R, Edwards R, et al. Aorticside branch embolization before endovascular aneurysm repair: incidence of type II endoleak. J Vasc Intervent Radiol 2001; 12:337–341.

18. Walker S, Macierewicz J, Hopkinson B. What happens to gelatin sponge treated AAA after endovascular grafting? On critical issues in endovascular grafting 1999, Malmö Sweden.

19. Görich J, Rillinger N, Sokiranski R, et al. Treatment of leaks after endovascular repair of aortic aneurysms. Radiology 2000; 215:414–420.

20. Gilling-Smith G, Brennan J, Harris P, Bakran A, Gould D, McWilliams R. Endotension after endovascular aneurysm repair: definition, classification, and strategies for surveillance and intervention. J Endovasc Surg 1999; 6(4):305–307.

21. White GH, May J, Petrasek P, Waugh R, Stephen M, Harris J. Endotension: an explanation for continued AAA growth after successful endoluminal repair. J Endovasc Surg 1999; 6(4):308–315.

22. Resch T, Lindblad B, Lindh M, Brunkwall J, Ivancev K. Aneurysm expansion and retroperitoneal hematoma after thrombolysis for stent-graft limb occlusion caused by distal endograft migration. J Endovasc Ther 2000; 7(6):446–450.

21

Sac Exclusion, Endopressure, and Endotension Following Endovascular Repair of Abdominal Aortic Aneurysm: The Role of Sac Volume Measurement

Mohan Adiseshiah
University College London Hospital, London, England

Successful and safe endolumenal repair (ER) of abdominal aortic aneurysms (AAA) and other aneurysms is routinely undertaken, but remains a controversial therapeutic choice in the context of standard open repair (OR). Until the results of properly conducted randomized controlled trials of these 2 types of surgery are known, only anecdotal and case series data are available for guidance to assist in selecting patients for each operation. The balance of evidence to date is that the < 30 day mortality is comparable in each case, but there are few hard data to judge which treatment is associated with lower morbidity. It is probable that the length of inpatient stay and speed of recovery is more favorable with ER (1).

What is not clear is how the treatments measure up to each other in the long term. It is established that there is an immediate 24% reported endoleak rate with most large series of ER (2). It is likely that type II and immediate type IV endoleaks probably seal spontaneously and do not require intervention. With regard to type I endoleakage, some will lead to sac expansion and rupture unless treated. However, although the total number of persistent type I endoleaks is estimated to be 5–15%, the number that will definitely cause sac rupture is unknown. Most worrying of all are those rare cases of sac expansion, due to presumed raised endopressure, which develop in the absence of obvious endoleakage of any type (3). As the sac volume increases in these cases, it is likely that there is an increase in endotension, which results in AAA rupture. Finally, cases of late endograft slippage or disruption will result in new endoleakage— type I or type III—which invariably result in sac expansion and rupture (4).

I. SAC EXCLUSION

Successful sac occlusion is usually judged by absence of flow outside the endograft within the sac, so-called *perigraft flow*. This is difficult to determine with certainty at completion angiography on the operating table. It is best determined by computed tomography (CT) with delayed pictures to detect type II endoleak. Properly validated duplex ultrasound in the hands of an excellent technologist also provides reliable evidence of endoleak or its absence.

Sac shrinkage usually follows successful sac exclusion (5). This is not evident until 6 months after surgery (see Fig. 1).

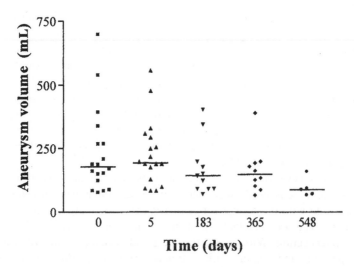

Figure 1. Column scatter graph showing the change in aneurysm volume after endografting with the Talent system. There is marked sac shrinkage with time. (From Ref. 5.)

In gross cases of shrinkage, there will be a diminution in maximum sac diameter. However, when sac shrinkage is less pronounced, only sac volume measurements will reveal the change (6). In a minority of cases, the sac will disappear altogether at approximately 1 year after surgery (Fig. 2).

In cases where preexpanded unsupported PTFE has been used for endograft construction, successful sac exclusion is not accompanied by sac shrinkage up to 5 years after surgery. However, no cases of AAA rupture have so far been reported.

II. ENDOPRESSURE

Little is known regarding sac pressure after successful or unsuccessful ER, especially over a period of weeks and months. Sac pressure data immediately following endovascular repair show a variable drop in pressure and a dampening of its waveform in comparison to systemic pressure (7,8). A fall to < 40 mmHg or to less than 50% of systemic pressure is probably compatible with successful sac exclusion. Unfortunately, there are no long-term data that allow correlation of sac size with the original sac pressure change immediately following ER. On the whole, provided a pressure drop as described above is observed along with a change from systemic pressure wave form to a more damped type of trace, successful sac exclusion can be expected.

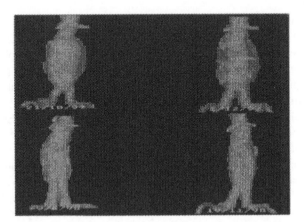

Figure 2. Three-dimensional reconstruction of AAA at 6-month intervals following ER with bifurcated Talent endograft. Note eventual disappearance of sac.

The ideal form of follow-up after ER would include sac pressure measurements on a continual basis. Unfortunately, the technology for these data is not available at the present time.

The alternative to endopressure measurement is sac volume measurement at the present time (9). Following ER, the sac volume increases slightly at day 5, probably because of the increase in sac thrombus. By 6 months a significant reduction in sac volume is detectable in the majority of cases treated by manufactured supported endografts. In the case of unsupported PTFE endografts, no further volume change occurs up to 5 years from ER.

With immediate persistent type I endoleak, the sac size remains unchanged or increases. If endoleak is detected at ER or soon after, we perform repeat spiral CT to look for persistence of endoleak and sac size increase at 6 weeks. If the sac does not increase in size, further observation is justified in the hope that the endoleak will close spontaneously. The finding of sac volume increase is an indication for further intervention to prevent the development of critical endotension and sac rupture. This involves pinpointing the site of endoleak by selective angiography and then secondary repair. In cases of late endoleak from endograft slippage or disruption (late type I, III, or IV endoleaks), there is an increase in sac volume, usually after a period of sac shrinkage or stable volume. Again, this is an indication for secondary intervention to prevent AAA rupture.

III. ENDOTENSION

This phenomenon occurs at the surface of the AAA sac. On an individual basis, if the tension reaches a critical value as a result of sustained high endopressure, AAA rupture occurs. The incidence of this complication is unknown, but is reported by EUROSTAR (10) as occurring < 1% per annum as a late phenomenon. This may be a conservative estimate due to underreporting and long-term deaths ascribed to other causes (11). This is the most dreaded complication of ER and is the major reason that ER has not replaced conventional open repair in geometrically suitable patients. Treatment of this condition carries a high mortality.

Endopressure secondary to untreated persistent immediate or late endoleak leads to this critical level of endotension. Currently, the best indication of the sustained endopressure is sac volume increase. Thus, sac volume increase constitutes an absolute indication for secondary intervention.

There are rare cases reported of rupture of the AAA, with or without demonstrable endoleak in the early postoperative period, i.e., < 30 days. In these cases there has been no increase in sac volume, probably because sufficient time had not elapsed to allow sac expansion. Further, it is possible that some part of the AAA may have suffered trauma and weakening of a landing site during deployment.

Finally, most sinister of all are those rare cases of sac rupture following sac expansion without evidence of endoleak (12). From animal experiments it has been shown that thrombus at a fixation site, while preventing endoleak, allows transmission of pressure into the sac (13). This could lead to critical endotension and then AAA rupture. Most cases reported occur months or years after ER and are confined to two commercially manufactured devices so far. It is likely that endograft disruption occurs without visible endoleak. This may produce occluding thrombus at the sites of graft failure, which then transmit systemic pressure into the sac leading to critical endotension and eventual AAA sac rupture.

IV. CONCLUSION

Endoleakage remains the Achilles' heel of ER. Its precise effects remain unknown. However:

1. Most immediate type II and some type I endoleaks will seal spontaneously within a few weeks.
2. Immediate type I endoleaks that cause sac volume increase should undergo secondary intervention. Those that do not cause sac volume increase may be observed for a longer time. (We intervene if they persist for more than 6 months even if there is no sac volume change.)
3. Late type I (endograft migration) and type III and IV endoleaks are associated with sac volume increase and should undergo urgent secondary intervention.
4. Sac volume increase without obvious endoleak is probably device related, is a sinister development, and should be treated by secondary intervention before critical endotension leads to AAA rupture.

REFERENCES

1. Zarins CK, White RA, Scawarten D, et al. AneurX stentgraft versus open surgical repair of abdominal aortic aneurysms: multicentre prospective clinical trial. J Vasc Surg 1999; 29:292–305.

2. Schurink GWH, Aarts NJM, van Bockel JH. Endoleak after stent-graft treatment of abdominal aortic aneurysm: a meta-analysis of clinical studies. Br J Surg 1999; 86:581–587.

3. White GW, Yu W, May J. Endoleak-proposed new terminology to describe incomplete aneurysm exclusion by an endoluminal graft (letter) [see comments]. J Endovasc Surg 1996; 3:124–125.

4. Lumsden AB, Allen RC, Chaikof EL, et al. Delayed rupture of aortic aneurysms following endovascular stent grafting. Am J Surg 1995; 170:174–178.

5. Singh Ranger R, McArthur T, Della Corte M, et al. The abdominal aortic aneurysm sac after endoluminal exclusion: a medium-term morphologic follow-up based on volumetric technology. J Vasc Surg 2000; 31:490–500.

6. Wever JJ, Blankenstein JD, Th MMW, et al. Maximal aneurysm diameter follow-up is inadequate after endovascular abdominal aortic aneurysm repair. Eur J Vasc Endovasc Surg 2000; 20:177–182.

7. Chuter T, Ivancev K, Malina M, et al. Aneurysm pressure following endovascular exclusion. Eur J Vasc Endovasc Surg; 13: 85–87.

8. Treharne G, Loftus IM, Thompson MM, et al. Quality control during endovascular repair: monitoring sac pressure and superficial femoral artery velocity. J Endovasc Surg 1999; 6:239–245.

9. Singh Ranger R, Adiseshiah M. Differing morphological changes following endovascular AAA repair using balloon—expandable or self expanding endografts. J Endovasc Ther 2000; 7:479–485.

10. Buth J, Harris PL. Endoleaks, endotension, sac morphology after endovascular AAA repair: What are the implications, based on the Eurostar results? VEITH 27th global, 2000.

11. Gilling-Smith GL, Martin J, Sudhindran S, et al. Freedom from endoleak after aneurysm repair does not equal treatment success. Eur J Vasc Endovasc Surg 2000; 19:421–425.

12. Fisher RK, Brennan JA, Gilling Smith GL, et al. Continued sac expansion with absence of endoleak is an indication for secondary intervention. Eur J Vasc Endovasc Surg 2000; 20:96–98.

13. Marty B, Sanchez LA, Ohki T, et al. Endoleak after endovascular graft repair of experimental aortic aneurysms: Does coil embolisation with angiographic "seal" lower intra-aneurysmal pressure? J Vasc Surg 1998; 27:454–462.

22

Opinions on Endoleaks and Endotension

Jan D. Blankensteijn
University Medical Center Utrecht, Utrecht, The Netherlands

Although the ultimate goal of endovascular aneurysm repair (EAR) is to prevent death from rupture, the primary objective of placing an endograft in an abdominal aortic aneurysm (AAA) is to exclude the sac from the circulation. Soon after the introduction of this new technique, a situation was recognized in which the exclusion was incomplete. Irrespective of the lack of understanding of the short- and long-term consequences of this condition, it seemed reasonable to consider it an undesirable outcome.

Today, over 10 years after the first human EAR, incomplete exclusion is called "endoleak" and several types are recognized. Although much experience has been gained, the consequences of an endoleak are still far from fully understood. As a matter of fact, several confusing observations in patients with and without endoleaks have been reported, which has led to much controversy. This chapter outlines the author's personal experiences and views on the issue of endoleak and endotension.

There are two core problems with the concept of endoleak as a measure of success or failure. First, endoleak does not equal failure. Spontaneous seal and subsequent aneurysm sac shrinkage is a well-recognized entity (1). Second, absence of endoleak does not equal success. Continued aneurysm growth and rupture without endoleak has been documented (2,3).

A large variation in reported endoleak rates of 2–70% also adds to the confusion (4). At least to some extent, missed endoleaks and misclassified endoleaks must be responsible for this. Presumably, differences in imaging quality from institution to institution explain a large proportion of this variation. Branches that maintain a patent connection with the aneurysm sac are not very difficult to identify. However, tracking these flow channels up or down to the sealing zones, in order to make the distinction between type I and type II, is much more likely to be dependent on the observer and the imaging modality and equipment used. It is conceivable that many of the reported type II endoleaks are in fact type I endoleaks in which the connection with the endovascular anastomosis has been missed. The incidence of true type II endoleaks may be very low. This theory provides an answer to the question why some branches stay open after EAR—because a connection (which may be difficult to visualize) exists with the main lumen.

Another point to make is that the AAA sac exclusion may well be relative instead of absolute. It is not unlikely that partial depressurization can cause one aneurysm to maintain its size or even grow, whereas another aneurysm in a similar pressure situation might shrink. This situation might even exist in a single patient in whom a certain pressure could lead to shrinkage of the sac in one area with concurrent localized expansion elsewhere (5).

Finally, the exclusion may be dynamic instead of static. As such, the sac may be completely excluded at one point in time but pressurized at another. For instance, with the patient in a supine position (on the CT-gantry), flow in the endoleak may come to a halt, while in a different body posture or during activity high endoleak flow rate may exist. The accepted theory describing the sequence of events in successful EAR starts with the exclusion of the aneurysm from the circulation, and the resulting pressure drop subsequently causes the remaining sac to shrink. Conceivably, the situation is more complex as almost all aneurysms have patent side branches preoperatively (1). Since most of the AAAs are decreasing in size in the first year after EAR, the preoperatively patent side branches appear to have no bearing on the success of the exclusion of the sac (6). How should this be explained?

Theoretically, immediately after the placement of an endovascular graft, a patent branch should be classified as a type II endoleak. Probably in the first minutes, maybe hours or days, retrograde flow into the sac will cease, leading to thrombosis at the ostium. This ostial thrombus appears to be able to isolate the sac from the arterial circulation. Otherwise EAR could not work.

If, for some reason, flow into or out of one or more side branches does not come to halt, it may show up as an endoleak postoperatively. In case of direct communication with a type I leak, chances of spontaneous closure of such a large flow channel are small. But also branch-to-branch communications may prevent a type II endoleak to thrombose. Continued flow through small channels in the otherwise excluded aneurysm sac or noncommunicating retrograde "puffs" of blood into the sac do not necessarily maintain pressures high enough to prevent the sac from shrinking. On the other hand, thrombosis of the side branch origin might not isolate the sac from arterial pressure from the lumbar and inferior mesenteric arteries. This phenomenon of pressure transmission through thrombus has been shown to be proportional to the diameter and length of the thrombosed side branch lumen (7). Based on those experimental data it was hypothesized that long and narrow side branches feeding endoleaks would be incapable of transmitting pressure, leading to sac shrinkage even if the flow channel remains patent. Large and short side branches, on the other hand, would lead to significant pressure transmission and subsequent sac growth, irrespective of the patency of the responsible channel.

To describe the situation of pressure, the term *endotension* has been proposed, meaning persistent or recurrent pressurization of the aneurysm sac after endovascular repair (8). With this definition the questionable assumption is being made that there will be situations after EAR with pressure and situations without. Based on the theory described above, it is more likely that a whole range of pressures can exist after EAR. If this is true, the endotension concept does not do much to describe success or failure, as it is unknown what magnitude of pressure would have to be called endotension.

There has been debate on whether to reserve the term endotension to describe pressurization of the sac in the absence of an endoleak (9). This discussion seems a little bit beside the point. Whether endoleak is included in the definition of endotension or not, the rationale for proposing the term endotension in the first place was sac growth without a detectable endoleak (3,8). As the definition is based upon "persistent or recurrent pressurization of the sac," patients with endotension but a shrinking sac can be expected, leading to even more confusion. If the definition of endotension would just address whether the sac is growing or not, simply describing size would suffice.

The term *endoleak* is necessary because it describes something for which no other term exists. If the aneurysm grows despite the (apparent) absence of an endoleak, there is some pressure in the sac. Pressure is a physical entity that can (and should) be measured—no other term is needed.

The next logical step would be to measure pressure in the sac as a parameter of successful exclusion (10). If this pressure could be monitored noninvasively using telemetry devices, all of the drawbacks of measuring volume or looking for endoleaks as described above could be bypassed. With current volume/diameter methods, at least two measurements more than 3–6 months apart are needed to prove that the exclusion is successful. It has been hypothesized pressure measurements could provide a single-instance measure of success. With the above-described potentially dynamic and relative nature of sac pressures, it is not hard to imagine pressure measurements having a significant number of false-positive and false-negative readings. Actually, some evidence exists that pressures might not be evenly distributed in an aneurysm after endograft placement. This would require several pressure transducers in the sac (5).

In conclusion, the presence or absence of endoleak cannot predict or fully describe the outcome after EAR, because accurate detection and classification of endoleaks is difficult with current imaging modalities. Conceivably, exclusion is relative and dynamic rather than absolute and static. Using both sac size changes (diameter but preferably volume) and pressure measurements, it should be possible to give the full picture. However, pressure probes cannot be expected to be the one and only follow-up modality. The ultimate measure of success remains to be defined. The concept of endotension only further confuses the issue.

REFERENCES

1. Broeders IA, Blankensteijn JD, Eikelboom BC. The role of infrarenal aortic side branches in the pathogenesis of endoleaks after endovascular aneurysm repair. Eur J Vasc Endovasc Surg 1998; 16(5):419–426.
2. Fisher RK; Brennan JA; Gilling-Smith GL; Harris PL. Continued sac expansion in the absence of a demonstrable endoleak is an indication for secondary intervention. Eur J Vasc Endovasc Surg 2000; 20(1):96–98.
3. Gilling-Smith GL, Martin J, Sudhindran S, Gould DA, McWilliams RG, Bakran A, et al. Freedom from endoleak after endovascular aneurysm repair does not equal treatment success. Eur J Vasc Endovasc Surg 2000; 19(4):421–425.
4. Schurink GW, Aarts NJ, van Bockel JH. Endoleak after stent-graft treatment of abdominal aortic aneurysm: a meta-analysis of clinical studies. Br J Surg 1999; 86(5):581–587.
5. Blankensteijn JD, Olree M, Mali WP, Eikelboom BC. Parameters of Successful Endovascular Repair of Abdominal Aortic Aneurysms. 4th International Workshop on Endovascular Surgery (abstr). Ajaccio, Corsica, France, June 1997.
6. Wever JJ, Blankensteijn JD, Th MMW, Eikelboom BC. Maximal aneurysm diameter follow-up is inadequate after endovascular abdominal aortic aneurysm repair. Eur J Vasc Endovasc Surg 2000; 20(2):177–182.
7. Ohki T, Veith FJ. Are all endoleaks equal? European Society for Vascular Surgery (abstr). London, UK. September 2000.

8. Gilling-Smith G, Brennan J, Harris P, Bakran A, Gould D, McWilliams R. Endotension after endovascular aneurysm repair: definition, classification, and strategies for surveillance and intervention. J Endovasc Surg 1999; 6(4):305–307.

9. White GH, May J. How should endotension be defined? History of a concept and evolution of a new term. J Endovasc Ther 2000; 7(6):435–438.

10. Baum RA, Carpenter JP, Cope C, Golden MA, Velazquez OC, Neschis DG, et al. Aneurysm sac pressure measurements after endovascular repair of abdominal aortic aneurysms. J Vasc Surg 2001; 33(1):32–41.

23

Complications of Endovascular Abdominal Aortic Aneurysm Exclusion: Evolving Concepts in Endoleak and Endotension

Christopher J. LeSar
Eastern Virginia Medical School, Norfolk, Virginia, U.S.A.

George H. Meier
Eastern Virginia Medical School and Norfolk Surgical Group, Ltd., Norfolk, Virginia, U.S.A.

The natural history of an untreated abdominal aortic aneurysm (AAA) is one of expansion, sometimes leading to rupture and death of the patient. The primary endpoint of any therapy must therefore address and alter this natural history to be successful. Conventional operative aneurysm resection and grafting is a durable surgical gold standard, but morbidities in this elderly population are generally high, and mortalities unavoidable. Endovascular therapy has engendered new excitement and promise for affecting the progression of abdominal aortic aneurysm expansion while reducing the need for traditional open repair (1).

In the early experience of endovascular aortic repair, residual blood flow outside of the endograft, but within the aneurysm sac, has been termed endoleak. This persistent flow has been noted to occur frequently, and most endoleaks are associated with branch vessels arising from the aortic aneurysm. In spite of the frequency of this event, the intra-aneurysmal blood flow along with the resultant pressure has not affected the success of this procedure. The aneurysm sac in the majority of endovascularly treated patients, despite endoleak, has stabilized or decreased in size (1,2). Despite general short-term success with aneurysm sac shrinkage, only time can determine the ultimate durability of this technique (3). It is, therefore, of utmost importance that long-term postoperative surveillance becomes standardized in this population. Surveillance by computed tomography (CT) and color duplex ultrasonography (CDU) has been utilized to determine the presence of endoleak, but the best modality and frequency of diagnostic study remains to be defined. Finally, the concept of endotension has been developed to describe the forces found within the residual aneurysm sac. Endotension, without evidence of endoleak, may result in AAA expansion secondary to these poorly understood forces.

I. ENDOLEAK

Incomplete exclusion of the aneurysm sac with ongoing residual flow outside of a successfully placed endograft has been termed "endoleak." Many different classification schemes have been developed defining endoleak in relation to the anatomical origins, the chronological time of onset, and the physiological characteristics of the source of flow (4). The most widely used classification defines endoleak from the anatomical origin of the flow. Type I endoleaks are associated with the attachment system, either proximally or distally. Type II endoleaks are from residual patent inferior mesenteric and lumbar vessels remaining within the aneurysm sac. Type III endoleaks are intrasegmental and are found only in modular devices where multiple components are utilized. Lastly, type IV endoleaks, or transgraft flow, occurs through defects in the fabric of the device. Of the two devices currently FDA-approved, the majority of the endoleaks have been type I and II (1–4).

The natural history of endoleak following endoluminal aneurysm repair has importance in defining the long-term success of this procedure. The ultimate goal of endograft placement is freedom from rupture, and this will rely on the forces that promote morphological changes within the aneurysm sac. Multiple opinions and considerable debate exist over the optimum management of endoleak (5–7). Direct arterial flow into the residual aneurysm sac from attachment site endoleaks (type I) has been considered clinically significant with early intervention for this problem the general consensus. Type III and IV endoleaks, as defined above, are rare entities, and individual assessment will direct either observation or treatment. Substantial controversy exists as to the appropriate course of management of patients with hemodynamically active, high-flow, branch vessel endoleaks (type II). Aggressive policies used to address type I endoleak have been employed by some to eliminate type II endoleaks, despite risk, discomfort, and cost. Other investigators have relied on observation and continued surveillance with the knowledge that AAA sac size usually decreases, even with an endoleak present (8). Although restraint may be warranted in patients with active type II endoleaks, safety demands aggressive surveillance at the very least.

These difficulties have led some investigators to undertake a careful physiological evaluation of endoleaks with CDU in order to delineate vessels involved, direction of flow, and to determine the waveform hemodynamics of these branch vessel endoleaks (8). Parent et al. (8) showed that with the type II endoleaks, two patterns of flow have been identified, each having very different waveform characteristics by ultrasound analysis. Type II endoleak flow patterns may have a "biphasic" or "monophasic" waveform suggesting inflow and outflow vessels. The majority of patients (7/10) with persistent type II endoleaks who exhibit this pattern have shrinking aneurysms. Three patients, however, experienced expansion requiring additional intervention, and these events reinforce the concept of sustained surveillance. The presence of a "to-fro" spectral Doppler signal found in a type II endoleak has a pattern similar to that observed in the neck of a femoral false aneurysm and is suggestive of a single vessel origin. Of importance, this "to-fro" pattern precedes endoleak closure in the majority (7/10) of these cases (9). The implication is that this Doppler velocity waveform may predict a benign course.

The nature of the coagulation and fibrinolytic systems acting within an endothelium-lined aneurysm sac should not be disregarded. Endoleaks have been shown by midterm results to have a dynamic nature (2,8,10). Type II endoleaks with "biphasic" flow patterns can become "to-fro" and then disappear. Also, persistent type II leaks with large channel "biphasic" flow patterns within the aneurysm sac have developed subsequent type I endoleaks. The vast majority of midterm data shows sac shrinkage leading to successful outcomes; however, the excluded aneurysm sac is in a state of flux. It is the individuals with late development of type I endoleaks and aneurysm sac enlargement, for unknown reasons, in whom surveillance and early intervention will hopefully prevent adverse outcomes.

Additional concerns pertaining to our understanding of endoleaks revolve around the "missed endoleak" and "misclassified endoleak." A small type I endoleak classified as a branch vessel leak may have serious implications; generally, type I endoleaks rarely thrombose and may get larger over time. Similarly, a missed endoleak may have significant clinical implications despite the amount of flow, or size of the leak, secondary to the active and changing nature of endoleaks. Routine aggressive surveillance is the only fallback in preventing endograft failure, leading to AAA sac enlargement with possible rupture.

II. ENDOLEAK DETECTION

The missed endoleak in patients with endovascular aneurysm repairs may be a more common problem than otherwise believed. The limitations of our technology to detect an endoleak as well as the practical aspects of data acquisition by our technologists cause difficulty. At our institution, the ideal test for endoleak detection is the combination of CT scanning with utilization of state of the art CDU technology. In our endograft experience, comparing all patients examined with both modalities, CDU has found twice as many type II endoleaks with verified flow as did contrast CT scanning using standardized protocols (8). High-flow type I endoleaks were detected by both tests, in all cases. This data is in direct contrast to the general opinion that contrast CT is the "gold standard" in detecting endoleak. In a study by Wolf et al., in which contrast CT and high-quality CDU exams were performed, they found that both exams were predictive in assessing endoleaks (11). An important distinction, however, must be made concerning the utilization of CT technology and the significant time that was invested in post-CT processing on a computer work station, rendering three-dimensional reconstruction, shaded surface displays, maximum intensity projections, and curved planar reformations. This technology, not routinely available in many centers, demonstrates the utility of a high-quality CDU exam for the detection of an endoleak. The concept that contrast CT, without the significant postprocessing, may detect only large endoleaks, secondary to limited resolution, remains an unproven but significant conclusion.

Although CDU can effectively identify the presence of endoleak, delineate vessels involved, detect direction of flow, and provide hemodynamic information not available by other testing modalities, newer technologies may further refine the detection of subtle endoleaks. Duplex assessment with ultrasound contrast may be the most sensitive test to date for determining low flow or small endoleaks (12). Although ultrasound contrast agents remain under investigation at our institution, two clinical cases currently support this hypothesis. In the first patient, the Ancure (unsupported) graft had significant wall motion, in phase with the cardiac cycle, during the CDU exam. This motion, in our experience, suggested the presence of an endoleak, which was not demonstrated by contrast CT. A prolonged CDU exam was performed

with an indeterminate result, but with the administration of Optison®
ultrasound contrast, the endoleak was detected in the area adjacent to the wall
motion after only an 80-second delay. This time delay implies that the
negative CT result may be related to the extreme delay in flow and that the
delayed acquisition sequence in the standard CT protocol was out of phase
with the delivery of sufficient contrast to the aneurysm sac. In the second
example, the patient experienced an iliac artery expansion and was
subsequently treated with a Wall stent to seal a presumed distal type I
endoleak. This iliac vessel failed to shrink in size over an extended time
despite CT and CDU negative exams. Ultrasound contrast demonstrated a
small type II lumbar endoleak with a "monophasic" waveform and with
careful scrutiny a very small area of flow along the iliac limb suggesting
residual or recurrent Type I endoleak. Both patients were clinically suspected
of harboring an endoleak, but demonstration required ultrasound contrast,
with confirmation by spectral waveform analysis, despite contrast CT and
extensive negative CDU exams. The ability of a test to document the presence
of endoleaks must have a specific inherent resolution below which the
detection of endoleaks is unattainable. We propose that the amount of flow in
the endoleak determines the success of detection, dependent on the inherent
resolutions of each testing modality (Fig. 1). It is our experience that high-flow
endoleaks are easily detected by all modalities and that low-flow endoleaks
can only be detected by CDU and ultrasound contrast alone.

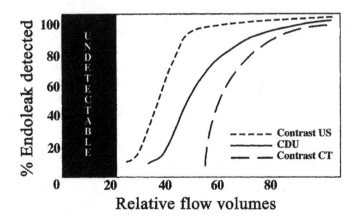

Figure 1. The detection of an endoleak depends on the ability of the test to
determine flow within the aneurysm sac. Very low flow volumes are likely to be
undetectable.

III. ENDOTENSION

Confounding definitions of "endotension" exist within the body of the literature, but this entity has been held responsible for not only aneurysm expansion but also rupture (13). Therefore, it is important to examine and determine what this entity is, how it functions, and why it exists. In 1999 Gilling-Smith proposed a new term, endotension, to define a new method of categorizing pressure rather than flow (endoleak) within the aneurysm sac. Endotension was defined as persistent or recurrent pressurization of the aortic aneurysm sac after endovascular repair. The system was stratified into three grades of endotension: grade I, harboring high-flow graft-related endoleak; grade II, low-flow branch vessel endoleak; and grade III, without endoleak (14). White narrowed the definition to mean "pressurization of the aneurysm sac after endovascular repair without evidence of endoleak," and despite Gilling-Smith's rejection of the change in this definition, endotension is currently viewed by most as sac expansion without endoleak (15).

Endotension resulting in AAA expansion can only be caused by physical forces acting on the residual aneurysm sac. These forces can be further defined as hemodynamic forces (e.g., missed endoleak) or nonhemodynamic static forces (of unknown origin). The current testing modalities (CT, ultrasound, and angiography) are the usual avenue for assessment of the aneurysm sac. However, the resolution of our testing is limited, and therefore a substantial number of false-negative exams could exist. Since even small endoleaks harbor systemic pressures, the expansion of an AAA sac without a demonstrable endoleak may lead to the false conclusion that endotension exists. In reality, missed endoleak, secondary to our inability to define small endoleaks, is the most likely explanation. Hemodynamic causes for endotension are more probable than "pressure trapping" nonhemodynamic endotension, although in theory this entity exists. Both PTFE and Dacron grafts have been noted to cause spontaneous perigraft seroma formation (16). If the grafts in some patients act as a highly selective filter, seroma formation within the hemodynamically excluded aneurysm sac could cause an increase in pressure.

Additionally, an extreme form of no flow endoleak can occur where an in-flow ball-valve–like effect results in "pressure trapping." This circumstance would be similar to the situation of a nonreversed saphenous bypass with an intact valve. Systolic pressure in the clamped vein graft would be found because the pressure is trapped downstream to the competent valve. The conduit would be nonpulsatile, the flow zero, and the maximum pressure would approach systolic pressure. Despite the theoretical ideas concerning endotension, the fact is that most expanding aneurysms with an unknown etiology which come to explant are often found to have evidence of endoleak, if not overt blood flow. (*Editor's Note:* This not always the case.)

Meier et al. performed a more definitive and exacting exploration for the presence of endotension in a large prospectively acquired study population with a high incidence of endoleak (17). The Ancure core lab data set, both well known and highly respected, allowed characterization of independently assessed imaging data with patients having abdominal aortic aneurysm exclusion over a 7-year period. In order to evaluate for endotension, three subpopulations of patients were subjected to analysis. Out of 476 patients evaluated, 144 (30%) met the strict criteria for never leaking (no endoleak) and represented the purest group in which endotension could be expected. If endotension were sporadic and truly a different physiology, then this group would be the most likely to exhibit endotension. The annualized change in AAA size was -5.2 mm/year in this group, and only two patients demonstrated aneurysm expansion greater than 5 mm. The next population in which endotension could potentially be present was in patients with sealed endoleaks after initial endoleak. All patients who had an initial endoleak and who were then without endoleak at any remaining time points were analyzed further. Transmission of pressure through the clot sealing the aneurysm sac has been one of the leading theories for endotension, as originally proposed by Gilling-Smith. In this group with sealed endoleak, 78 (16.4%) of 476 patients had an annualized change in AAA size of -5.8 mm/year, with no patient expanding greater than 5 mm. The last group that was studied had late endoleak development where endotension could have led to aneurysm expansion and subsequent endoleak formation. If these patients had a significant size increase in the residual sac prior to the development of the endoleak, then endotension might have been responsible. In this late endoleak group, 41 (8.6%) of 476 patients had an annualized change in AAA size of -1.4 mm/year, and three patients experienced greater than 5 mm expansion. All three patients had technically inadequate early imaging exams on further review. Therefore, this study concluded that in all subpopulations who were likely to harbor endotension, only five patients experienced greater than 5 mm expansion, and the majority of these patients were found to have poor imaging studies. We contend that nonhemodynamic endotension is a rare entity at best, and endotension, in most cases, represents missed endoleak.

IV. CONCLUSIONS

Endovascular therapy has been successful in altering the natural history of abdominal aortic aneurysm expansion. Intense surveillance of the excluded aneurysm in order to obtain long-term data is still needed to know the true consequences of endoleak and its effect on the durability of endograft therapy. The ability to detect endoleaks is of paramount importance; CDU and Doppler ultrasound contrast are sensitive means to detect this complication. After an extensive review of a large prospective endograft trial, no evidence of significance AAA expansion was seen in the absence of endoleak defined by appropriate imaging studies. In our opinion, aneurysm sac expansion without overt endoleak commonly represents "missed endoleak" and should be evaluated by intensive imaging prior to attributing any aneurysm sac changes to endotension.

REFERENCES

1. Zarins CK, White RA, Moll FL, Crabtree T, Bloch DA, Hodgson KJ, Fillinger MF, Fogarty TJ, et al. The AneuRx stent graft: four-year results and worldwide experience. J Vasc Surg 2001; 33(2):S135–S144.
2. Makaroun MS. The Ancure endografting system: an update. J Vasc Surg 2001; 33(2):S129–S134.
3. Rhee RY, Eskandari MK, Zajko AB, Makaroun MS, et al. Long-term fate of the aneurysmal sac after endoluminal exclusion of abdominal aortic aneurysms. J Vasc Surg 2000; 32(4):689–696.
4. Wain RA, et al. Endoleaks after endovascular graft treatment of aortic aneurysms: classification, risk factors, and outcome. J Vasc Surg 1998; 27(1):69–80.
5. Marty B, Sanchez LA, Ohki T, Wain RA, Faries PL, Cynamon J, Marin ML, Veith FJ. Endoleak after endovascular graft repair of experimental aortic aneurysms: Does coil embolization with angiographic "seal" lower intraaneurysmal pressure? J Vasc Surg 1998; 27(3):454–462.
6. Gorich J, Rilinger N, Sokiranski R, Kramer S, Schutz A, Sunder-Plassmann L, Pamler R. Embolization of type II endoleaks fed by the inferior mesenteric artery: using the superior mesenteric artery approach. J Endovasc Ther 2000; 7:297–301.
7. Makaroun M, Zajko A, Sugimoto H, Eskandari M, Webster M. Fate of endoleaks after endoluminal repair of abdominal aortic aneurysms with the EVT device. Eur J Vasc Endovasc Surg 1999; 18:185–190.
8. Parent N, Meier GH, Godziachvili V, LeSar CJ, Parker FM, Carter KA, Gayle RG, DeMasi RJ, Marcinczyk MJ, Gregory RT. The incidence and natural history of Type I and II Endoleak: a 5-year follow-up assessment by color duplex ultrasound. J Vasc Surg 2002. In press.
9. Carter KA, Nelms CR, Block PH, Gregory RT, Parent FN, DeMasi RJ, Meier GH, Gayle RG. Doppler waveform assessment of endoleak following endovascular

repair of abdominal aortic aneurysm: predictors of endoleak thrombosis. J Vasc Tech 2000; 24(2):119–122.

10. Zarins CK, White RA, Hodgson KJ, Schwarten D, Fogarty TJ. Endoleak as a Predictor of outcome after endovascular aneurysm repair: AneuRx multicenter clinical trial. J Vasc Surg 2000; 32(1):90–107.

11. Wolf YG, Johnson BL, Hill BR, Rubin GD, Fogarty TJ, Zarins CK. Duplex ultrasound scanning versus computed tomographic angiography for postoperative evaluation of endovascular abdominal aortic aneurysm repair. J Vasc Surg 2000; 32(6):1142–1148.

12. Heilberger P, Schunn C, Ritter W, Wber S, Raithel D. Postoperative color flow duplex scanning in aortic endografting. J Endovasc Surg 1997; 4:262–271.

13. Gilling-Smith GL, Martin J, Sudhindran S, Gould DA, McWilliams RG, Bakran A, Brennan JA, Harris PL. Freedom from endoleak after endovascular aneurysm repair does not equal treatment success. Eur J Vasc Endovasc Surg 2000; 19(4):421–425.

14. Gilling-Smith G, Brennan J, Harris P, Bakran A, Gould D, McWilliams R. Endotension after endovascular aneurysm repair: definition, classification, and strategies for surveillance and intervention. J Endovasc Surg 1999; 6:305–307.

15. White GH, May J, Petrasek P, Waugh R, Stephen M, Harris J. Endotension: an explanation for continued AAA growth after successful endoluminal repair. J Endovasc Surg 1999; 6(4):308–315.

16. Blumenberg RM, Gelfand ML, Dale WA. Perigraft seromas complicating arterial grafts. Surgery 1985; 97(2):194–204.

17. Meier GH, Parker FM, Godziachvili V, Demasi RJ, Parent FN, Gayle RG. Endotension after endovascular aneurysm repair: the Ancure experience. J Vasc Surg 2001; 34(3):421–426.

Index

Treatment, University of California at
San Francisco, 139
Type II endoleaks
Buenos Aires experience, 95, 98,
99
catheter embolization, 211–220
clots, 20
coil embolization, 153
completion arteriograms, 226
Consensus Questionnaire results,
8–9, 13–15, 17
definition, 26, 27, 28, 30, 31,
125–126, 260
device instability, 136
endotension case studies, 69
EUROSTAR series, 48, 172
IMA as backflow source, 221–235
intraoperative, 202, 205, 206
known, aneurysm rupture, 136–137
late, 32–33
limited pressure increase, 112
Liverpool definition, 102
Malmö perspective, 241–245, 253
Nottingham perspective, 170–174,
178–180
ostial thrombosis, 256
percutaneous embolization, 37
prevention, 12
rates, 170
secondary procedures, 231
SMA, 148
spiral computed tomography, 139
Stanford University (California)
study, 121
treatments, 127, 140, 151–153
Zenith stent-graft, 243–244
Type III endoleaks
case study, 65–66
classification, 14
Consensus Questionnaire results, 8
definitions, 26, 27, 28, 31, 102, 126,
260
EUROSTAR series definition, 48
intraoperative, 202, 205, 206, 210

[Type III endoleaks]
Liverpool definition, 102
Malmö perspective, 253
Nottingham experience, 174
spiral computed tomography, 139
treatments, 129, 154–156
University of California at San
Francisco, 141
Vanguard endograft, 96, 97
Type IV endoleaks
classification, 14
coil embolization, 156–157
definition, 26, 27, 28, 126, 260
endoleak source location, 33–34
intraoperative, 200, 205, 206
Liverpool definition, 102
Malmö perspective, 253
Nottingham experience, 175
protective thrombus, 137
spiral computed tomography, 139
treatments, 129, 156–157
Zenith endoluminal stent-grafts,
86
Type V endoleaks
classification, 14
type A, 21, 22
type B, 21, 22
type C, 21, 22
type D, 21, 22

Ultrasound (*see* Color duplex
ultrasound)
Uni-iliac stent-graft, intraoperative
aortogram, 240, 241
University of California at San
Francisco, 135–142
University College London Hospital,
249–254
University of Pennsylvania Medical
Center, 199–210, 221–235
University of Pennsylvania School of
Medicine, 125–33, 140
University of Pittsburgh Medical
Center, 185–98